Preface

Three years ago the Standing Committee of Members of the Royal College of Physicians devised a series of annual conferences entitled 'Interfaces in Medicine'. Designed to bring general practitioners and physicians together, the first was on cardiovascular disease and the second on asthma. For the third, the subject of diabetes could not be bettered. This lifelong disorder taxes the skill and tolerance of both kinds of doctor as well as nurses, dieticians, chiropodists, other experts and also, of course, the patient.

The two sides, hospital and general practice, have moved much closer together in the last decade. GPs have taken a larger role and some now run their own mini-clinics. Diabetes specialist nurses are now universally appreciated and most of us cannot understand how we ever managed without them. Hospitals have reached out from their base by creating diabetes centres with dedicated staff. Patients have the convenience of open access, small rooms and informal atmosphere. Compare this with large hospital clinics, open for perhaps half a day a week, where patients wait on benches for hours before seeing a new doctor for just a few minutes.

In terms of patient satisfaction the service has greatly improved in recent years. Could this trend, to take the service to the patient, be extended further? Is there still a place for the specialist hospital unit? A few years ago some GPs thought not, but this is not true today. We all recognise the real difficulties of treating some diabetics, especially insulin-takers and, above all, children and adolescents. The stakes are now also too high to adopt an easy-going attitude towards complications which can be devastating or even fatal. With greatly improved methods of treating complications, such as retinopathy and nephropathy, we need to screen patients for their early signs.

The proceedings of this conference encourage us towards the necessary synthesis of all types of diabetes care which well-informed patients now expect.

David Pyke
Registrar
Royal College of Physicians

Editors' introduction

This book looks at several of the current themes in the care of diabetes at the present time. We have reached a point where anxieties about the effects of new legislation are being tackled by both professionals and patients, all keen to get on with the job in hand. Many problems still to be faced are addressed in this book. John Ward begins with an overview of the current provision of care in the UK. Diabetes care, to be effective and to give consumer satisfaction, has to be well organised. The consumer needs to be actively involved in this process, learning about the modern management of diabetes and thus knowing what minimum standards of care to accept. These issues are clearly argued by Stephen Tomlinson who also shows in Chapter 2 how audit can be used as a powerful tool for improving care.

GPs have always been involved in the care of diabetes, looking after perhaps the majority of such patients. The GP's role is now changing, with greater emphasis on the provision of a system of care and more detailed involvement in management. Michael Hall describes in Chapter 3 how GP referral patterns to specialists will vary according to the resources available and emphasises the special relationship between GP and patient which should always be preserved.

Non-insulin dependent diabetes has been regarded, traditionally, as a mild condition with simple therapeutic needs. Unfortunately, as Robert Tattersall points out in Chapter 4, it is anything but mild, causing substantial morbidity and mortality. It must surely be a target for greater endeavours towards preventive care. Two areas where such preventive care might be fruitful are the common problems of obesity and hyperlipidaemia. In the absence of intervention studies in diabetics, Peter Kopelman recommends strategies for the primary care management of these conditions based upon clear cut objectives and the efficient use of practice resources. Diabetes would cause little concern if it did not result in progressive degradation of health. Andrew Boulton reviews the range of diabetic complications and indicates the attention to detail necessary to prevent them or to delay and minimise their consequences.

The use of insulin has tended to become more specialised and complex. GPs may wish to become more involved in this form of therapy because of the increasing number of elderly diabetics who eventually come to need it. Felix Burden provides an introduction to the subject and Diana Piper illustrates in Chapter 8 how insulin treatment can be started at home with minimal disruption to life style.

Ultimately, the aims of diabetes care are to improve the quality and quantity of life. It is perhaps easy for the health care team to get carried away by the process of care and by the impact of patient behaviour on audit figures. What the patient wants is a happy life. George Alberti argues that it should be possible to have both successful management of diabetes *and* a happy life. Achieving this apparently simple objective requires endeavour and expertise from patients and professionals alike.

The papers in this book are derived from an 'Interfaces in Medicine' symposium held at the Royal College of Physicians in February 1991. A pleasing theme throughout the symposium was the increasing integration of modern diabetes care. General practice and hospital teams are achieving this by redefining standards and by working more closely together.

Ian Lewin
Carol Seymour

Contributors

K. G. M. M. Alberti DPhil FRCP *Professor of Medicine, The Medical School, Newcastle upon Tyne.*

Andrew J. M. Boulton MD MRCP *Senior Lecturer in Medicine, University of Manchester Medical School; Honorary Consultant Physician, Manchester Royal Infirmary.*

A. C. Burden MD FRCP *Consultant Physician, Leicester General Hospital; Honorary Senior Lecturer, Leicester University Medical School.*

Michael S. Hall BSc MB BS D Obst RCOG FRCGP *Senior Lecturer in General Practice, University of Exeter Postgraduate Medical School; Principal in General Practice, Bow, Devon.*

Peter Kopelman MD MRCP(UK) *Senior Lecturer in Medicine, The Royal London Hospital; Consultant Physician, Newham General Hospital, London.*

Diana Piper RGN *Diabetes Specialist Nurse, Northern Devon Healthcare, Barnstaple, Devon.*

Robert Tattersall MD FRCP *Professor of Clinical Diabetes, University Hospital, Nottingham.*

Stephen Tomlinson MD FRCP *Professor of Medicine, University of Manchester Medical School; Honorary Consultant Physician, Manchester Royal Infirmary and The Manchester Diabetes Centre.*

John D. Ward BSc MD FRCP *Consultant Physician, Royal Hallamshire Hospital, Sheffield; Chairman, Patient Services Advisory Committee, British Diabetic Association.*

Contents

1 | Provision of diabetes care in the UK

John D. Ward
Royal Hallamshire Hospital, Sheffield

There have been marked improvements in diabetes care in the UK in the last 20 years. The number of consultant diabetologists has increased and the diabetes specialist nurse has been introduced as a clinical practitioner and educator. These developments have been coupled with more integrated involvement of dieticians and chiropodists and the setting up in many districts of dedicated diabetes centres. These advances have taken place without financial incentive, without hasty ill-conceived bureaucratic plans and without encouragement to develop a competitive attitude to the provision of medical care. They have occurred because of the ideals of the professionals involved and because of the pressure from the British Diabetic Association (BDA) for adequate facilities and standards of care.

During this time, GP involvement in diabetes care has increased significantly and this has been mostly successful.[1,2,3] The Royal College of General Practitioners has set up vocational training schemes in general practice, which have undoubtedly increased knowledge and understanding of diabetes. Recent changes in the pattern of general practice seem to have encouraged more GPs to take on diabetes care, but not always for the correct reasons. With thought, consideration and collaboration, integrated diabetes services can be developed which will lead to even further improvements in the quality of care. Traditional views from hospital and general practice may need to be modified, but if excellent standards of care for all diabetics are the primary goal there should be every chance of success.

Hospital and general practice care

For many years, diabetes care has been provided either in large hospital based diabetic clinics or in general practices near to patients' homes. Many patients now attend both these services as part of a shared care system. With hospital based diabetes care, the emphasis is on team work involving highly trained individuals backed up by good facilities. The team might consist of: senior physician and junior doctors, specialist nurses, chiropodist, dietician, orthoptist, psychologist and manager. There is close liaison with other specialists such as: obstetrician, renal physician and ophthalmic, vascular and orthopaedic surgeons. In many instances diabetologists carry out combined clinics with such experts. Thus, the provision of diabetes care is essentially organisation of team members so that patients have ready access to the various specialties when needed. Within this context it is often possible to give considerable professional time to problems which arise at short notice, such as the unco-operative adolescent, worries about complications, impotence or erratic control.

Hospital based diabetic clinics do have potential disadvantages. For some patients, hospitals are large, threatening places and often some distance from home. Even so, many people are willing to make the journey if services are of sufficient quality. Traditionally, a fault of the hospital diabetic clinic has been the large size, the excessive waiting time and the tendency for patients to see a different junior doctor at each visit. Dr Pat Thorn from Wolverhampton, the pioneer of diabetes mini-clinics once said: 'If I had diabetes I would not go to my own clinic.' It is good that such 'cattle market' clinics are being improved by careful thought and organisation. District diabetes centres[4] have helped to solve such problems. They can provide a permanent focus for patients, offering education, advice, support and identification of early complications. They can also provide an environment for collaboration between GPs, hospital doctors and others involved in diabetes care.

Some hospital based professionals seem to fear that the new arrangements in general practice will encourage GPs to reduce substantially their demand upon hospital services. However, the transfer back to general practice of patients not needing hospital care will allow specialised resources to be concentrated upon those who really need them. At the present time it also seems likely that 25% of diabetics receive no formal care. Identifying and providing care for this group will itself take up much general practice time.[5] Now and for the future, we should be collaborating with each other to offer appropriate resources to each patient.

General practice diabetes care is often highly convenient for patients, being close to home and more personal than hospital care. It is usually less threatening than hospital and less costly. However, it is difficult to build an expert diabetes team for every general practice although dieticians and chiropodists could be funded and shared by a number of practices. Anyone giving diabetic advice needs adequate training. Thus, the nurses in general practice should measure up to the same level of education as diabetes specialist nurses who have worked in diabetes units, attended English National Board nursing courses and other educational sessions. It is certainly unfair to expect a practice nurse with little knowledge of diabetes to start running a diabetic clinic in the community.

It is often assumed that the GP has ample time to spend with patients but this is frequently not the case because of pressure from other duties. The GP diabetes service therefore has to be well organised to respond to the unexpected needs of people presenting with complicated problems. If such a service is based on a local diabetes centre, the necessary time can often be found even at short notice.

A major responsibility for those setting up diabetes care is the provision of continuing education for patients and their carers. This must be far more comprehensive than the distribution of a few educational leaflets. Services should consist of individual teaching sessions, group sessions and the use of audio visual aids. The educational programme should not be confined to diet and insulin injection technique but should include coping and self-care strategies, awareness and prevention of complications and foot care. Unless those who aim to provide a diabetes service can also offer this comprehensive educational programme they should not enter the field of diabetes care.

Interface between hospital and general practice

Hospital and general practice need to agree upon how diabetes care should be shared. Each group should be clear about what it offers and which patients it prefers to see. This will undoubtedly vary from district to district and from practice to practice. Some GPs might wish to offer comprehensive care to all non-insulin dependent diabetics but might prefer eye examinations to be done by another agency such as a hospital clinic, a retinal camera service or an optician. It seems likely that many insulin dependent diabetics, those difficult to control and those with complications, will tend to be seen more often in hospital, but this should be agreed by the two parties. A co-operation card should be a mandatory part of the diabetic service, so that each party involved in care knows exactly what other parties are doing.

A local steering committee should be established to organise diabetes services in a community. This should consist of:

- an FHSA administrator;
- the FHSA independent medical adviser;
- a GP from the local medical committee;
- the diabetologist;
- the local diabetes specialist nurse;
- a Health Authority representative and;
- a patient member of the local BDA branch.

This committee should agree the protocols for diabetes care in hospital and general practice, collaborate with the many other agencies essential for good diabetes care and arrange for local audit of care.

Central to planned diabetes care is the concept of a computerised register which could be held in the district diabetes centre. Every diabetic in a defined area should then be registered as attending a hospital clinic, a GP clinic or both and this entry should be updated at each annual review.

Contracts

A major fear for the future centres around the suggestion that diabetes services will be subject to contracting arrangements. 'Purchaser and provider' are euphemisms for the obvious buying and selling that is proposed. Many involved in diabetes care feel that attempts at buying and selling within the complexities of this condition will result in muddle and chaos. It is worrying to feel that referral to a specialist diabetes service might depend upon the balance of a GP's budget. Freedom for patients to move between general practice and hospital must be allowed as frequently as necessary according to clinical circumstances. It is unrealistic to define a contractual number of clinic visits per year. Some patients might need no more than an annual review whilst others might need urgent referral followed by weekly visits because of control problems or complications. It is also difficult to fit the convenience and flexibility of district diabetes centres into an exact costing system. Patients often call in for advice, education and support, without the knowledge of their GPs. Such patients may not be attending any other formal diabetes care service.

Financial constraints reducing the flexibility of diabetes care might well result in barriers which would ultimately work against patients' best interests. If there are no such barriers, collaboration between general practice and hospitals can continue to progress. If health authorities insist on buying and selling diabetes services, specific situations should be identified and costed as accurately as possible. The following categories might be looked at:

1. New patient requiring insulin therapy: full educational programme including dietary advice, injection technique and monitoring strategies; clinical assessment; home visits, support and frequent attendances over 3 months.
2. New patient not requiring insulin: full educational programme including dietary advice and monitoring strategies; clinical assessment; home visits, support and frequent attendances again over 3 months. A patient requiring a change to insulin therapy should be regarded as a new category 1 patient.
3. Patient with known insulin dependent diabetes with no problems attending once or twice a year for general care, plus detailed examination to identify risk factors.
4. Special groups:
   a. Diabetic pregnancy or gestational diabetes;
   b. Patients assessed as having risk factors, eg for foot ulceration;
   c. Adolescence where flexibility and prolonged counselling time are necessary;
   d. Impotence where special services and expertise are required;
   e. Patients with advanced complications in several tissues;
   f. Re-referral of established diabetic patients with new problems.

Conclusion

Great improvements in diabetes care have taken place in the UK in the past 20 years. Recent changes in the National Health Service have stimulated a change in the pattern of care with an increase in the number of people involved who can give more time and expertise to patients and their problems. There is the opportunity for greater collaboration between hospital and general practice and any attempt at commercial control of patient movement which impedes this should be resisted. Stringent assessment of the quality and outcome of services will be necessary in all areas so that standards of diabetes care continue to rise throughout the next decade.

References

1. Thorne PA, Russell RG. Diabetic clinics today and tomorrow: mini-clinics in general practice. *Br Med J* 1973; **ii**: 534–6.
2. Hill RD. Community care for diabetics in the Poole area. *Br Med J* 1976; **i**: 1137–9.
3. Day JL, Humphreys H, Alban-Davis H. Problems of comprehensive shared diabetes care. *Br Med J* 1987; **294**: 1590–2.
4. Day JL, Spathis M. District diabetes centres in the United Kingdom. *Diabetic Med* 1988; **5**: 372–80.
5. MacKinnon M. The role of nurses in general practice. *Pract Diabetes* 1986; **3**: 232–4.

2 | The aims of diabetes care

Stephen Tomlinson
Department of Medicine, University of Manchester

Diabetes is common, affecting 1–2% of the population. About 20% of people with diabetes are insulin dependent (Type 1) and about 80% are non-insulin dependent (Type 2). The incidence of Type 1 diabetes is highest in the age group 0–20 years and then appears to be constant from the age of 20 to the age of 75 years. On the other hand, the incidence of Type 2 diabetes increases with age but the majority of patients acquire diabetes before the age of 55 years. There is some evidence that the prevalence of both types of diabetes is increasing. Furthermore, it has been suggested for Type 2 diabetes that there are as many undiagnosed cases as those known to have the condition. In some groups, such as Asians over 60 years old, the prevalence of diabetes may be as high as 25%. High quality medical care needs to be extended to all of these people to enhance both the quality and the quantity of life.

Complications of diabetes

Both types of diabetes cause a great increase in morbidity and mortality. For Type 1 diabetics at the age of 30 there is a tenfold increase in relative mortality and for Type 2 diabetics diagnosed in their fourth decade there is an age related reduction in life expectancy of ten years. Fortunately, there is some evidence that at least in Type 1 diabetes mortality rate is beginning to fall. In one study of patients with Type 1 diabetes, the relative mortality decreased by more than 40% during the period from 1933 to 1972.[1,2]

Cardiovascular disease is extremely common in diabetics and this largely accounts for their excess mortality. Overall the incidence of fatal and non-fatal coronary artery disease is up to three times higher than in non-diabetics, this increase being greater in younger age groups and particularly marked in women. It is the leading cause of death in Type 1 diabetes, accounting for 40–60% of all deaths. Type 2 diabetes is particularly associated with potent risk factors for the development of cardiovascular disease including hypertension, lipid disorders and smoking.[3,4]

Renal failure is another important cause of morbidity and mortality. A decade ago, diabetic nephropathy accounted for almost 20% of deaths in diabetics under the age of 50 years. Currently, up to 40% of people with a ten year history of Type 1 diabetes develop renal impairment. The presence of proteinuria is itself a poor prognostic sign, even before the development of end stage renal failure, the median survival from onset being only 7–8 years.[5] Cardiovascular diseases cause death in 25–40% of people with Type 1 diabetes who also have proteinuria.[6] Nephropathy is also an important cause of morbidity in Type 2 diabetes. Up to 50% of all patients on renal replacement therapy have Type 2 diabetes and these same people are also at high risk of coronary heart disease and amputations.[4]

Other major complications of diabetes are only too familiar. Neuropathy and peripheral vascular disease lead to a fifteen-fold increase in the risk of gangrene and lower limb amputation. Diabetes is probably the commonest predisposing factor for elective lower limb amputation.[7,8] Impotence is present in 50% of men over the age of 40 with Type 1 diabetes. Diabetes is the commonest cause of blindness in the working population and the risk of blindness is ten-fold that of the non-diabetic.[9] The incidence of congenital malformations in the infants of mothers with Type 1 diabetes is increased three- to four-fold[10] and up to 50% of women with gestational diabetes will ultimately develop Type 2 diabetes. Added to all these causes of morbidity and mortality are the enormous social consequences of diabetes. People with newly diagnosed Type 1 diabetes have their driving licences temporarily revoked, those already stabilised on insulin cannot follow certain occupations and insurance premiums are often heavily loaded. Diabetes can disrupt families. In health economic terms diabetes costs up to one billion pounds per annum in the United Kingdom.[11,12]

What can we do?

A primary aim of treatment is the relief of symptoms of hyperglycaemia. This should be associated with improvements in the quality of life in the short and the long term. A second major aim is the prevention of chronic complications of diabetes and thus a reduction in avoidable excess mortality. For Type 1 diabetes these complications are related to duration of the disease. However, as

many as 25–50% of people with Type 2 diabetes have complications
at first presentation but again the incidence increases with time
from diagnosis. There is now good evidence that the microvascular
complications of diabetes, neuropathy, retinopathy and nephropathy, are associated with poor glycaemic control. This is probably
also true for Type 2 diabetes but additional factors are also important here such as hypertension, obesity, lipid disorders and
smoking.[13,14,15] In both types of diabetes one of the aims of treatment
is therefore to improve glycaemic control. Even so, this should not
be achieved at the expense of reduced quality of life resulting from
increased risk of hypoglycaemia.

Whilst improved glycaemic control may ultimately prevent some
of the complications, another aim of treatment should be their early
detection since there is good evidence that prompt intervention can
prevent or delay deterioration. This is certainly true for diabetic
retinopathy and is probably true for nephropathy associated with
hypertension. Furthermore, appropriate patient education following the early detection of neuropathy might not only prevent re-
current foot ulceration, but also reduce the risks of amputation.[16]

Patient education and diabetes

Effective patient education can enhance quality of metabolic
control, improve the safety of treatment, increase social and psychological well being, reduce complications and reduce costs. A North
American study showed that educational programmes associated
with structured care can substantially reduce admissions and length
of stay in hospital. Episodes of diabetic ketoacidosis were cut to a
quarter and the number of amputations was halved.[17,18] These
educational programmes for patients and their relatives depend
upon diabetes specialist nurses who have played such a major role
in the great changes that have occurred in diabetes care in the last
two decades. In the year following the appointment of a diabetes
specialist nurse in central Manchester almost a hundred people
with newly diagnosed insulin dependent diabetes were initially
treated and stabilised at home, thus saving almost £200,000 on inpatient costs. The appointment of a nurse to implement educational programmes in diabetes footcare has been associated with a
reduction of 40% in the number of amputations over a period of
two years. It therefore seems clear that educational programmes can
have a major impact on morbidity and quality of life in the short
term and an even greater impact in the long term.

Audit in diabetes care

Audit is primarily a mechanism for addressing and improving the quality of patient care, enhancing medical education and identifying ways of improving efficiency.[19] In reviewing how audit might be implemented it is worth outlining some of the features which are involved. Three main interrelated categories of clinical care can be measured: *structure* (quantity and type of resources available); *process* (what is done to the patient, eg measurement of blood pressure) and *outcome* (result of clinical intervention). Audit should include:

- recorded observation of practice;
- establishment of standards or targets;
- comparison of observed practice with set standards;
- implementation of change and observation of the impact of change.

It should be educational and relevant to patient care; it should be performed by clinical peers with voluntary participation and it should be set locally by participating clinicians. In addition audit should be non-threatening, interesting, objective and repeatable. Ideally it should also be simple, cheap and cause minimal disturbance.[19] Medical audit is not a management tool and its objective is not directed towards cutting costs but it may identify more efficient ways of using resources, thus leading to better and also cheaper patient care. Once changes have been made, aimed at improving the quality of patient care, they should be re-evaluated by the same process. The true value of audit lies in the useful action which results.

Patient register and minimum standards of care

A starting point for audit in diabetes could be the establishment of a patient register. This might include age, sex and type of diabetes. The aim should then be to develop a more comprehensive register to include details of treatment such as insulin, oral hypoglycaemic agents and diet alone. The next element might be to define minimum standards of care for each patient including annual or more frequent review of symptoms, weight, lying and standing blood pressure, visual acuity, examination of fundi through dilated pupils and examination of feet for pulses and vibration perception. Biochemistry should be audited annually both individually and on a group basis by looking at serum creatinine, glycated haemoglobin (HbA1) or fructosamine, cholesterol and triglycerides. Annual audit of urine tests should include detection of proteinuria and, in selected cases, microalbuminuria.

Audit of activity and avoidable outcomes

The quantity of care supplied to individuals and groups of diabetic patients easily lends itself to audit. In addition to assessing delivery of care within a practice, GPs might also wish to analyse the annual number of hospital outpatient and inpatient episodes generated by their patients. This approach can be used to monitor potentially preventable outcomes such as foot ulcers, amputations, renal replacement treatment, laser therapy and problems of pregnancy. It has allowed us to identify individual episodes of diabetic keto-acidosis in central Manchester and to devise strategies to reduce the hospital admission rate.

It is important to assess individual outcomes such as death and stroke because of the clinical lessons which may be learnt. However, the small number of cases per general practice per annum may not be sufficient for meaningful statistical analysis. One way of dealing with this is for several practices to undertake joint audit of pooled data for selected problems. This would have additional benefits from an educational point of view, especially if undertaken in collaboration with the local diabetes team at the district general hospital.

Consumer satisfaction

Evaluation of any clinical service should include patients' perceptions and expectations. In the past, certainly in inner city hospitals, these expectations have been unduly low through lack of education. For example, in one survey of the traditional diabetic clinic at the Manchester Royal Infirmary, 85% of patients waited longer than one hour to see a doctor for an average consultation time of five minutes. They believed that routine checks had been performed on their kidneys in 20%, their feet in 30%, their heart and circulation in 50% and their eyes in 55% of cases. Curiously, 15% did not appear to realise that they had come to have their diabetes checked. Even so, when asked for their opinion, 65% were satisfied with the level of service received. It is hoped that the days of the traditional diabetic clinic are numbered, as hospitals are now improving their standards of care by restructuring clinics or by establishing district diabetes centres.[20]

It is now appreciated that patients should understand in detail what minimum standards of care to expect. When this is achieved it becomes possible to make a meaningful assessment of the quality of service available. A simple and useful way to do this is to use a brief anonymous questionnaire seeking views on the comparison between a general practice mini-clinic and a hospital clinic. These questionnaires should first be given a trial with members of staff and then with a small number of patients, to ensure that questions are comprehensible and unambiguous. They might address topics such as clinic opening and waiting times, privacy, duration of consultation, environment, clinical care, information and education. Once questionnaires have been validated they can be applied repeatedly to the diabetic population over a period of time and the results used to adapt services to patients' needs.

The concept of consumer satisfaction should also operate at a professional level between the hospital service and general practice. Each should seek the views of the other about the quality of service provided. Again, simple questionnaires can produce useful information. Communication difficulties are often highlighted, such as inaccessibility of key individuals, delayed response to telephone calls and poorly constructed letters. Rapid access to information is essential for everyone involved in diabetes care and local solutions to these problems need to be found.

Setting targets

If targets for diabetes care are to be reached by a specific date they should be readily achievable and not at the limits of feasibility. Establishing targets for the structure and process of care might be the simplest way to start. Thus it might be reasonable to aim for identification of all patients on insulin and oral hypoglycaemic agents within one year and all people with diabetes irrespective of treatment within two years. Depending upon the number of mini-clinics to be held within a year, it might be feasible to establish a target such that 50% of people on the register would have seen the GP and practice nurse by the end of a year and perhaps 25% would also have seen a dietician and chiropodist. Subject to achievement, these targets might be reviewed and modified.

With regard to outcome measures, targets for weight reduction might be set for those with a body mass index greater than 28. Similarly, targets for improved glycaemic control might be set for all people with Type 2 diabetes. Thus if the mean HbA1 were initially 11% the aim might be a reduction to 10% within two years but with review at one year. Targets for blood pressure could be set for hypertensive and normotensive patients, specifying the frequency of measurement and the levels of pressure considered acceptable. Other clinical indices of quality of care could include diabetes related hospital admissions with the aim of reducing avoidable episodes.

Education for professionals

Patient education is an essential component of any diabetes service. Health care professionals delivering this also require their own educational programmes. Many need advice on what to teach and how to teach it, whether on a one to one or a group basis. Regional Health Authorities and Family Health Service Authorities (FHSAs) need to be aware of this so that they can make suitable provision. The rapid changes in diabetes care also create a need for regular local updates in addition to the intensive one-off programmes such as the English National Board 928 course for nurses. Courses for GPs, nurses, dietitians, chiropodists and other health professionals need to be co-ordinated so that the contents are appropriate without unnecessary duplication. Perhaps this is best done at a district level with guidance from the British Diabetic Association. District diabetes care steering groups which include consultants, GPs, specialist nurses, practice nurses, dieticians, chiropodists and the FHSA medical adviser might have a role in promoting this aspect of diabetes care.

Conclusion

Improvements in diabetes care are related to successful teamwork involving both the professionals and the patient. Exciting opportunities now exist for making measurable progress with greater emphasis on integration, co-ordination and partnership in the delivery of high quality care for people with diabetes.

References

1. Borch-Johnsen, K. IDDM. Incidence, complications, prevention with special reference to the impact of nephropathy. *Giornale Italiano di Diabetologia* 1990; **10**: 13–20.
2. Borch-Johnsen K, Kreiner S, Deckert T. Mortality of Type 1 (insulin dependent) diabetes mellitus in Denmark: A study of relative mortality in 2930 Danish Type 1 diabetic patients diagnosed from 1933 to 1972. *Diabetologia* 1986; **29**: 767–72.
3. Garcia MJ, McNamara PM, Gordon T et al. Morbidity and mortality in

diabetes in the Framingham population. Sixteen-year follow up study. *Diabetes* 1974; **23**: 105–11.
4. Gries FA. NIDDM - Prevalence, incidence, complications, prevention. The impact of arteriosclerotic complications. *Giornale Italiano di Diabetologia* 1990; **10**: 21–5.
5. Anderson AR, Christianson, JS, Anderson JK, Kreiner S, Deckert T. Diabetic nephropathy in Type 1 (insulin dependent) diabetes: An epidemiological study. *Diabetologia* 1983; **25**: 496–501.
6. Borch-Johnsen K, Kreiner S. Proteinuria value as predictor of cardio-vascular mortality in insulin dependent diabetes. *Br Med J* 1987; **294**: 1651–4.
7. Boulton AJM, Knight G, Drury J, Ward JD. The prevalence of diabetic neuropathy in an insulin treated population. *Diabetes Care* 1985; **8**: 125–8.
8. Most RS, Sinnock P. The epidemiology of lower extremity amputation in diabetic individuals. *Diabetes Care* 1983; **6**: 87–91.
9. Tomlinson S. Diabetes and its complications. *Seminars in Ophthalmology* 1987; **2**: 1–3.
10. Fuhrmann K, Reiher H, Semmler K et al. Prevention of congenital malformations in infants of insulin dependent diabetic mothers. *Diabetes Care* 1983; **6**: 219–33.
11. Gerard K, Donaldson C, Maynard AK. The cost of diabetes. *Diabetic Med* 1989; **6**: 164–70.
12. Williams R, Leing W. The health care costs of diabetes. *Giornale Italiano di Diabetologia* 1990; **10**: 99–101.
13. Pirart J. Diabetes mellitus and its degenerative complications: A prospective study of 4,400 patients observed between 1947 and 1973 (in three parts). *Diabete Metabolisme* 1977; **3**: 97–107, 173–82, 245–56.
14. Raskin P, Rosenstock J. Blood glucose control and diabetic complications. *Ann Int Med* 1986; **105**: 254–63.
15. Reaven GM. Role of insulin resistance in human disease. *Diabetes* 1988; **37**: 1595–1607.
16. Dahl-Jorgensen K, Brinchmann-Hansen O, Hanssen KF *et al.* Effect of near normoglycaemia for two years on progression of early diabetic retinopathy, nephropathy and neuropathy: The Oslo Study. *Br Med J* 1986; **293**: 1195–9.
17. Laugharne E. Tri-hospital diabetes education centre: The cost effective co-operative venture. *The Canadian Nurse* 1977; **September**: 14–9.
18. Miller LV. More efficient care of diabetic patients in a county hospital setting. *N Engl J Med* 1972; **286**: 1388–91.
19. *Medical audit: a first report.* London: Royal College of Physicians, 1989.
20. Day JL, Johnson P, Rayman G, Walker R. The feasibility of a potentially 'ideal' system of integrated diabetes care and education based on a day centre. *Diabetic Med* 1988; **5**: 70–5.

3 | Which diabetics need hospital follow-up?

Michael S. Hall

Department of General Practice, University of Exeter

Ultimate responsibility for care of diabetic patients living at home rests with the GP. Patients are registered with GPs and not with hospital consultants or diabetes centres. The contract is between the GP, the FHSA and the patient. GPs provide the greatest quantity of diabetes care in terms of numbers but some patients will also take part in shared care schemes with hospital clinics; others will occasionally receive most of their care from hospital units. The degree to which an individual diabetic needs hospital follow-up will depend very much upon the services provided by the primary care teams and the hospitals within a given locality. At the present time these services are undergoing a process of rapid evolution with the promise of a systematic improvement in the quality of care provided.

Locality plan for diabetes care

Unfortunately, in many parts of Britain the care for people with diabetes is poorly structured.[1,2,3] Most GPs and many hospital departments have yet to organise care in a way that ensures regular surveillance, covering a range of important checks for such patients. The quality of care is influenced by numerous factors, including:

- attitudes of GPs and consultants;
- support from nursing staff;
- facilities available;
- waiting lists;
- the distance individual patients live from their local centre.

Good diabetes care requires an agreed plan suited to local needs in which all those involved have a defined role. For the plan to succeed the participants must own and take responsibility for it by working together to design it. Putting together such a plan may be quite hard work. GPs, consultants, nurses and others involved must meet together. They need to find out what care is currently available before they can identify how to improve it. Striking a balance between what is desirable and what is achievable is not always easy. to ensure that patients receive a satisfactory standard of care one needs to construct a system which:

- identifies the GP's diabetic patients;
- utilises the strengths of individual practices;
- has a built in fail-safe recall system, and;
- co-operates with specialist units.[4,5]

The Exeter Diabetic Project enabled us to work on these problems.[6] We adopted the philosophy that all patients should expect regular surveillance provided by either a member of the primary health care team or by a member of the hospital team. 'What diabetic care to expect', the British Diabetic Association (BDA) charter for patients[7] accorded with our views and also served as a reminder that well-informed patients can take an active role in maintaining professional standards.

We have tried to encourage practices to adopt a care strategy based upon three principles advocated by Hurwitz:[8]

 i. identify all diabetic patients;
 ii. agree to follow the local care protocol, and;
iii. agree a simple annual audit of care.

A diabetic protocol was agreed between GPs, practice nurses and other practice staff together with the hospital based diabetes team of diabetologist, diabetes specialist nurse and ophthalmologist. This initiative was supported by the local medical committee. A patient-held co-operation card was also devised to encourage liaison between carers, patients and relatives. It is designed to show at a glance those procedures not yet completed in any 12-month period. It works reasonably well and has been slightly modified over three years to suit changes in practice.

The Exeter Diabetic Project continues to grow, providing support and also a regular newsletter for those working in diabetes care. The service will soon be linked to the district diabetic register allowing all participating GPs to take part in comparative local audit.

Who does what?

From the patient's point of view it is important that all the components of a surveillance check are carried out regularly and competently. As long as standards of care can be guaranteed it should not matter whether such procedures take place in general practice or in hospital. Consistent standards should make it possible for patients to receive care wherever they find it most convenient.

Practice nurses are now greatly involved in diabetes care, providing an important amount of the total care within general practice. There is clearly a need to ensure that, working in such a responsible area, they have appropriate training.

Which patients need to go to hospital?

It is often assumed that most insulin dependent diabetics attend hospital units and that most non-insulin dependent diabetics are cared for within general practice. Our district audit of all known diabetics in 160 out of 186 practices showed otherwise. Of the 2762 patients, 71% were under the sole care of their GP and this included 25% of insulin dependent diabetics.[9] These data reinforce the need to design appropriate diabetes services, recognising that primary care must continue to do much of the work.

Given that practices will provide different services for their diabetic patients, there will be a fairly large group who need hospital follow-up for tests such as annual ophthalmoscopy. Apart from those, there are other categories which need specialist care. These include: diabetes in childhood; newly diagnosed insulin dependent diabetes; diabetes in pregnancy; acute and chronic complications of diabetes.

It is always helpful for children with diabetes to have regular hospital follow-up. Whether this takes place in a diabetic clinic, diabetes centre or paediatric department will depend upon local arrangements. It is also important that they are offered regular support by their GP. The role and personal relationship of the GP needs to be understood by patient and parents and seen as a positive contribution. For example, GP and practice nurse could regularly complete a growth chart.

Patients with newly diagnosed insulin dependent diabetes benefit from hospital referral and initial follow-up. Some patients and GPs might prefer otherwise, in which case their alternative arrangements would need to meet the same standards of expertise and care, including access to the diabetes specialist nurse and dietician. If there is a local diabetes centre its educational resources could be offered when appropriate.

Undoubtedly *all* diabetic women who are pregnant or who are planning a pregnancy need referral both to the diabetes specialist unit and to the obstetric unit. Successful outcome of pregnancy has been shown to depend very much upon ideal control of diabetes and hence every possible effort should be made to achieve this. Again, the GP and primary health care team should continue to play their part in regular diabetes and antenatal care.

Acute complications of diabetes often require hospital referral. Illnesses like influenza or bronchitis may seriously upset glycaemic control and infective gastroenteritis with vomiting, diarrhoea and electrolyte disturbance may cause critical illness if not treated promptly in hospital. Patients whose diabetes is brittle or difficult to control often have personal problems. Sharing care of this group not only temporarily relieves the GP of a burden but sometimes provides real help. Often it is not a doctor who gives most support to this sort of patient but the practice nurse and the diabetes specialist nurse working together.

Hospital follow-up is most helpful for patients in whom complications have been detected at regular surveillance checks. Included in this group are those with difficult hypertension, albuminuria, microalbuminuria, sight threatening retinopathy, painful neuropathy, mononeuropathy and amyotrophy as well as those suffering from deteriorating feet or pre-gangrene and those with special problems such as impotence.

Continued involvement of the primary care team

Although patients may be referred to hospital for specific problems or long-term management they should be encouraged to maintain a good relationship with their own practice so that shared care can continue successfully. The primary care staff should fulfil their own part of the contract of care, supervising the prescription of treatment and encouraging compliance. The co-operation card should be checked to confirm that items of surveillance are carried out or organised by the hospital. This should occur at each contact between the patient and the practice even if the consultation is not about diabetes. This opportunistic approach often succeeds with patients who are unenthusiastic about keeping their routine surveillance appointments.

Conclusion

The BDA's leaflet for patients[7] says: 'The control of your diabetes is important, and so is the detection and treatment of any complications. Make sure you are getting the medical care and the education you need to ensure you stay healthy.' The primary health care team plays a key role in this process which also includes working cordially with colleagues in specialist units.

Acknowledgement

The Exeter Diabetic Project has depended upon the co-operation of all members of the team. The two research fellows, Dr Jonathan Stead and Dr Simon Dudbridge, were largely responsible for creating the goodwill and enthusiasm which enabled the scheme to work.

References

1. Yudkin JS. The quality of diabetic care in a London health district. *J Epidemiol Community Health* 1980; **34**: 277–80.
2. Hayes TM, Harries J. Randomised controlled trial of routine hospital clinic care versus routine general practice care for Type 2 diabetes. *Br Med J* 1984; **289**: 728–30.
3. Day JL, Humphreys H, Alban-Davies H. Problems of comprehensive shared diabetes care. *Br Med J* 1987; **294:** 1590–2.
4. Gibbins RL, Saunders J. How to develop diabetic care in general practice. *Br Med J* 1988; **297**: 187–9
5. Kopelman P, Keable-Elliott D. An inner city district diabetic care scheme. *Diabetic Med* 1990; **7**: 558–61.
6. Stead JW, Dudbridge SB, Hall MS, Pereira Gray DJ. The Exeter diabetic project: an acceptable district-wide education programme for general practitioners. *Diabetic Med* 1991; **8**: 866–9.
7. British Diabetic Association. What diabetic care to expect. *Diabetic Med* 1990; **7**: 554.
8. Hurwitz B. Getting Started on Diabetic Care. *Practitioner* 1987; **231**: 1525–31.
9. Hall MS. Diabetes: towards better care. *Practical Diabetes* 1990; **7**: 155–6.

4 | Non-insulin dependent diabetes: a wolf in sheep's clothing

Robert Tattersall

The University Hospital, Nottingham

Fifteen years ago I received from an insurance company a form asking 'Is the proposer a mild, moderate or severe diabetic?' Not knowing how to answer I phoned the medical officer who was surprised at my lack of understanding. In the language of Humpty Dumpty, words are what you choose them to mean, neither more nor less. 'Mild' evidently meant diet treated, 'moderate' meant tablets and 'severe' indicated insulin injections! My reply was that the severity of a disease should be judged by its consequences and not by the perceived complexity or unpleasantness of treatment, but this fell upon deaf ears. My aim is to explain that non-insulin dependent (NIDDM) and mild diabetes are not equivalent. To avoid a litany of unpleasant complications I shall try to tame the wolf by suggesting how the worst effects of NIDDM can be prevented or mitigated.

Prevalence

NIDDM is common and in all societies its prevalence increases with age, inactivity and body weight. For example, in the USA the prevalence is 4.3% in white women aged 45–54 years, rising to 8.9% in those aged 65–74. In most other racial groups NIDDM is even more common, affecting 7.5% of black women aged 45–54 years and 10.8% of those aged 65–74 years.[1] Indians in their homeland or after migration to the UK, Fiji or Mauritius have a four-fold higher prevalence than Caucasians.[2] The record is held by the Micronesian island of Nauru and the Pima Indians of Arizona where diabetes is epidemic. It affects nearly half the population over age 35 and leads to the typical complications.

Morbidity and mortality

Mortality from diabetes is consistently underestimated in official statistics. This is because it is under-reported by about 60% on the death certificates of older people with cardiac or cerebrovascular disease or multiple chronic conditions.[3] In a large cohort study of patients with NIDDM, 44% had died within 10 years and the excess mortality was already seen in the first year after diagnosis.[4] Excess mortality declined with increasing age at diagnosis so that those developing NIDDM over age 75 had a similar life expectancy to the general population. Nevertheless, the consequences of hyperglycaemia can be increasingly serious with advancing age. The mortality from ketoacidosis and hyperosmolar coma is 4.3% for those under 50 and rises to 43% in patients who are older.[5]

Patients with NIDDM use two to three times more hospital bed days than non-diabetics[6] and for some complications, particularly foot ulcers and amputations, the average hospital stay is six to seven times greater than for non diabetics of the same age. Hyperglycaemia also complicates diagnosis and management in older patients. For example it is often difficult to be sure whether urinary symptoms are due to infection, hyperglycaemia, prostatism or prolapse.

The major causes of death in NIDDM are myocardial infarction and stroke. Patients admitted with heart attack or stroke also have an increased prevalence of undiagnosed diabetes. Diabetic men are twice, and diabetic women three times as likely to die of myocardial infarction as their peers.[7] Most studies show a doubling of hospital mortality of NIDDM patients after myocardial infarction compared to non diabetics, the majority dying of pump failure. There is also an excess of heart failure in ambulant patients with NIDDM which cannot be explained entirely by ischaemic heart disease and which is probably due to diabetic cardiomyopathy.[8] Nevertheless, the main cause of mortality in NIDDM is ischaemic heart disease which, together with hypertension, is present in approximately half at the time of diagnosis of diabetes.[9]

The cause of the increased liability to heart disease is uncertain but several other metabolic abnormalities are found in addition to hyperglycaemia: hyperinsulinaemia, high serum LDL cholesterol and triglycerides, low HDL cholesterol, hypertension and central obesity. All are atherogenic as independent variables. Reaven has suggested that NIDDM may not be a specific disease entity but an expression of a more general disorder in which multiple metabolic abnormalities are caused by insulin resistance.[10] If this hypothesis is correct large vessel disease should not be categorised under the traditional umbrella of late complications since atherosclerosis and NIDDM would develop coincidentally, in parallel, or even in reverse sequence. It seems clear that 'the future strategy against premature mortality in NIDDM requires multifactorial approaches. At present we are doing too little too late, if anything can be done at all'.[11] We assume that treating hypertension and hyperlipidaemia in NIDDM will improve survival but we may need to start before the onset of hyperglycaemia.

The burden of complications in NIDDM

All GP lists will have at least one multicomplicated patient with NIDDM who requires care from several specialists. I can give an example of one of my own cases, a man with a previous history of duodenal ulcer at the age of 50. When he first presented with NIDDM at the age of 60 he already had background retinopathy, peripheral neuropathy and hypertension. Two years later he developed neuropathic foot ulceration and soon afterwards his retinopathy became proliferative and required laser therapy. Now at the age of 65 he has suffered a myocardial infarction and he has proteinuria.

A community study in Oxfordshire emphasised the extensive morbidity amongst diabetic patients over age 60 and the fact that complications were not confined to a single subgroup.[12] Of the 193 patients, 80% had developed diabetes below the age of 70. Treatment was with diet alone in 24%, diet plus tablets in 54% and insulin in 22%. Glycaemic control was generally poor with a median haemoglobin A1 of 9.7% (range 4.9–17.1%; normal range 5–7%). Symptomatic macrovascular disease, neuropathy and retinopathy were each present in a quarter of cases; visual impairment was present in a third and hypertension in half. Only 20% were free from complications of diabetes; 75% were also suffering from at least one other disease. The microvascular complications were as frequent as in younger patients but macrovascular disease and co-morbidity were much more common. One patient in ten was receiving no formal diabetic care, 25% had unmet chiropody needs and 80% on oral hypoglycaemic agents were taking either chlor-propamide or glibenclamide whose potential for causing serious or fatal hypoglycaemia is not sufficiently appreciated.[13]

Microvascular complications (retinopathy, nephropathy and neuropathy) in NIDDM are as common as in insulin dependent diabetes (IDDM) but much more likely to be present when diabetes is first diagnosed.[14] Hence a comprehensive clinical examination is especially important in newly diagnosed NIDDM.

Retinopathy

A major difference between NIDDM and IDDM is that retinopathy
is present in over a quarter of patients in the former category when
diabetes is first diagnosed.[15] Patients with NIDDM are more likely
to have maculopathy than the proliferative retinopathy of IDDM.
To detect maculopathy at a treatable stage such patients need
ophthalmoscopy and measurement of visual acuity at presentation
and then annually thereafter. They should be referred to an
ophthalmologist before visual acuity has fallen below 6/12. Some
very characteristic heartsink patients have the eye-foot syndrome.
These are usually middle-aged men who present with large neuropathic foot ulcers and deteriorating vision due to advanced
retinopathy. They appear unconcerned about both complications
and their mean survival is only five years.[16]

It is uncertain whether blood glucose control prevents progression of established retinopathy but there is no doubt that photocoagulation prevents visual loss in maculopathy, especially if applied
when patients still have good vision.[17]

Nephropathy

Persistent Albustix-positive proteinuria, the hallmark of established
diabetic nephropathy, develops in about 10% of patients known to
have NIDDM for over 10 years. Effective antihypertensive treatment
is the best way of slowing the inevitable decline in renal function.
Renal artery stenosis is common in hypertensive NIDDM patients[18]
and unsuspected bilateral disease carries the risk of acute renal
failure if angiotensin converting enzyme inhibitors are used.
Calcium channel blockers therefore seem most suitable, particularly
as they do not adversely affect blood glucose or lipids.

Many patients die from myocardial infarction or the consequences of fluid overload before their serum creatinine rises
above 700 μmol/l, the stage at which dialysis would usually be
considered.[19] Even so, NIDDM account for 11–84% of patients on
renal replacement programmes.[20, 21] The decision as to whether
these multicomplicated middle aged patients should be offered
such arduous and expensive treatment is often very difficult.

Feet

Middle-aged or elderly people with NIDDM are often divorced from
their feet, unable to see them because of poor eyesight, unable to

feel them because of neuropathy and unable to bend down to touch them because of arthritis. Superimposed on the vulnerability to pressure ulceration or other forms of trauma from neuropathy is the almost inevitable co-existence of peripheral vascular disease. This combination of risk factors accounts for the very high frequency of foot ulcers, infections and gangrene. Foot lesions account for 20% of hospital admissions in patients with NIDDM and in our unit the average stay for foot patients is over a month. Many or even most foot lesions are preventable and effective co-ordinated programmes of foot care can reduce the amputation rate by 50% or more. The famous American diabetologist, Elliot Joslin, put it well when he said (1934): 'It may seem a detail to tell patients to wipe their feet gently, but if you wish to avoid gangrene you must enter into all these minutiae'. *Co-ordinated footcare* has to include identifying feet at risk by palpating foot pulses and testing sensation then educating patients and relatives, stressing the potential dangers and explaining what to do if a problem arises. Regular chiropody and suitable footwear have to be provided.

Conclusion

The Oxford survey showed that 80% of NIDDM patient over age 60 had complications.[12] This study alone illustrates the scale of the problem and gives the lie to the idea that these people have mild diabetes and that they will be all right as long as they keep taking the tablets. It has been said that:

> People with diabetes should receive the best medical care available which in general requires a team approach ... it is the practitioner's responsibility to see that diabetic patients have the knowledge and skills necessary for self care and to ensure that hypertension, retinopathy, nephropathy and foot disease are diagnosed in a timely manner and treated appropriately.[22]

Since the average health district with a population of 250,000 contains about 3000 diabetics it was obvious, even before the White Paper, that most would have to be looked after by their general practitioners. To avoid the preventable disasters outlined in this paper all diabetics in a practice should be identified and a 'contract' drawn up for their care. Some will be appropriately looked after in their own practice whilst others will benefit from the expertise available in a hospital unit.

References

1. Harris MI, Hadden WC, Knowler WC, Bennett PH. Prevalence of diabetes and impaired glucose tolerance and plasma glucose levels in US population aged 20–74 yr. *Diabetes* 1987; **36**: 523–34.
2. Simmons D, Williams DRR, Powell MJ. Prevalence of diabetes in a predominantly Asian community: preliminary findings of the Coventry Diabetes Study. *Br Med J* 1989; **298**: 18–21.
3. Tattersall RB. Diabetes in the elderly—a neglected area? *Diabetologia* 1984; **27**: 167–73.
4. Panzram G, Zabel-Langhennig R. Prognosis of diabetes mellitus in a defined population. *Diabetologia* 1981; **20**: 587–91.
5. Gale EAM, Dornan TL, Tattersall RB. Severely uncontrolled diabetes in the over-fifties. *Diabetologia* 1981; **21**: 25–8.
6. Damsgaard EM, Froland A, Green A. Use of hospital services for elderly diabetics: the Frederica study of diabetic and fasting hyperglycaemic patients aged 60–74 years. *Diabetic Med* 1987; **4**: 317–22.
7. Gwilt DJ, Pentecost BL. The heart in diabetes. In: Natrass M ed. *Recent Advances in Diabetes*. London: Churchill Livingstone. 1986: 177–94.
8. Fisher BM, Frier BM. Evidence for a specific heart disease of diabetes in humans. *Diabetic Med* 1990; **7**: 478–89.
9. Uusitupa M, Siitonen O, Aro A, Pyorala K. Prevalence of coronary heart disease, left ventricular failure and hypertension in middle-aged, newly diagnosed type 2 (non-insulin-dependent) diabetic subjects. *Diabetologia* 1985; **28**: 22–7.
10. Editorial. Type 2 diabetes or NIDDM: looking for a better name. *Lancet* 1989; **i**: 589–91.
11. Panzram G. Mortality and survival in type 2 (non-insulin-dependent) diabetes mellitus. *Diabetologia* 1987; **30**: 123–31.
12. Neil HAW, Thompson AV, Thorogood M, Fowler GH, Mann JI. Diabetes in the elderly: the Oxford Community Diabetes Study. *Diabetic Med* 1989; **6**: 608–13.
13. Ferner RE, Neil HAW. Sulphonylureas and hypoglycaemia. *Br Med J* 1988; **296**: 949–50.
14. Watkins PJ, Grenfell A, Edmonds M. Diabetic complications of non-insulin-dependent diabetes. *Diabetic Med* 1987; **4**: 293–6.
15. Owens DR, Volund A, Jones D et al. Retinopathy in newly-presenting non-insulin-dependent (Type 2) diabetic patients. *Diabetes Research* 1988; **9**: 59–65.
16. Walsh CH, Soler NG, Fitzgerald MG, Malins JM. Association of foot lesions with retinopathy in patients with newly diagnosed diabetes. *Lancet* 1975; **i**: 878–80.
17. British Multicentre Study Group. Photocoagulation for diabetic maculopathy: a randomised controlled clinical trial using the Xenon arc. *Diabetes* 1983; **32**: 1010-16.
18. Renal artery stenosis in hypertensive diabetic patients. Ritchie CM, McIlrath E, Hadden DR, Weaver JA, Kennedy L, Atkinson AB. *Diabetic Med* 1988; **5**: 265–7.
19. Patterson AD, Dornan TL, Peacock I, Burden RP, Morgan AG, Tattersall RB. Causes of death in diabetic patients with impaired renal function: an audit of a hospital diabetic population. *Lancet* 1987; **i**: 313–6.

20. Berisa F, McGonigle R, Beaman M, Adu D, Michael J. The treatment of diabetic renal failure by continuous ambulatory peritoneal dialysis. *Diabetic Med* 1989; **6**: 67–70.
21. Grenfell A, Bewick M, Parsons V, Snowden S, Taube D, Watkins PJ. Non-insulin-dependent diabetes and renal replacement therapy. *Diabetic Med* 1988; **5**: 172–6.
22. The Carter Center of Emory University. Closing the gap: the problem of diabetes mellitus in the United States. *Diabetes Care* 1985; **8**: 391–406.

5 | Obesity and hyperlipidaemia in the non-insulin dependent diabetic patient

Peter Kopelman

The Royal London Hospital and Newham General Hospital, London

Obesity and hyperlipdaemia are well recognised accompaniments of diabetes mellitus and are well worth treating seriously. General practice health promotion activities, including diabetic clinics, offer a fresh opportunity to look at the management of patients with these conditions, allowing a preventive approach to care. This chapter looks at obesity and hyperlipidaemia related to non-insulin dependent diabetes and considers treatment strategies in the primary care setting.

Obesity

Measurement of obesity

Body mass index (BMI) has been adopted as a convenient measure of obesity and with the new GP contract it is now recorded in patients' notes. It is calculated by dividing body weight in kg by the square of the height measured in metres, though in many practices it will be calculated automatically by computer. Acceptable ranges are 20.1–25.0 for men and 18.7–23.8 for women.[1]. Obesity has been defined in various ways but indices of 27 for men and 25 for women correspond fairly closely to an excess of 20% above desirable body weight.

A further clinically useful index of obesity is the waist-to-hip ratio (WHR), comparing truncal with femoral-gluteal fat distribution. In moderate obesity this is more sensitive than BMI as a predictor of coronary heart disease (CHD)[2] and ideally should be measured in all diabetics with a BMI between 25 and 30. The patient should be standing for the measurements and breathing normally. Waist circumference should be taken at the mid-point between the lower rib margins and the anterior superior iliac spines; hip circumference should be measured at the widest level of the hips.[3] As a guideline, the WHR should be less than 0.94 in men and less than 0.83 in women.

Risks of obesity

Moderate and severe obesity are associated with progressive morbidity and mortality independent of age.[1,4] There is a strong relationship between obesity and the risk of CHD in both sexes. Thus, in men below the age of 75 mortality from cardiovascular disease increases in an almost linear fashion with increments in weight.[5] In non-diabetic women with a BMI greater than 29 the risk of myocardial infarction is increased three-fold compared to a normal weight group.[6] Diabetes magnifies this problem so that in diabetic women with a similar degree of obesity the risk is increased twelve-fold.

Upper body (truncal) obesity is associated with an increased risk of CHD. In one study the WHR was the most powerful predictor of the level of HDL2, a subfraction of HDL cholesterol generally associated with a reduced risk of CHD. Higher WHRs correlated with lower HDL2 levels.[7] This may partly explain why some non-insulin dependent diabetics (NIDDMs) with Syndrome X, consisting of insulin resistance, upper body obesity, hypertension and dyslipidaemia, are particularly at risk of CHD.[8] Those at highest risk are the severely obese, with a BMI greater than 30, and the moderately obese with upper body fat distribution as indicated by a WHR greater than 0.95.

Obesity in diabetic clinics

Despite the advances in diabetic therapy during the past 50 years, there has been no change in the prevalence of obesity in patients attending hospital diabetic clinics.[9,10] Typically, BMI will be greater than 25 in 50% of men and 66% of women. It will exceed 31 in 11% of men and 25% of women.[11] An average general practice will contain approximately 100 diabetic patients with an equal sex distribution and it is likely that almost all of those invited to attend a GP mini-clinic will be overweight to some degree. New approaches will be necessary to tackle this problem.

Team approach to treatment

The team approach to obesity works well in the primary care setting where the familiar environment encourages co-operation. Patients and their families need to look upon attendance at the clinic as an essential part of diabetes management. The practice nurse is crucial for the successful running of the health promotion clinic, but substantial input is required from the doctors and also a dietician and psychologist if available.

Principles of dietary strategy

Weight loss of 10–16% of initial body weight improves glycaemic control[12] and more substantial weight loss may also reduce morbidity and mortality from the atherosclerotic complications of diabetes. The success of a weight losing programme is related to the dietary prescription, the importance attached to it and the way in which it is communicated to patients, families and carers. Restriction of calorie intake is essential to ensure weight reduction. It may not be possible to define an ideal weight for a patient. However, a target weight should be negotiated at an early stage which is potentially attainable considering personal factors, the degree and duration of obesity and the outcome of previous weight losing regimens. The European NIDDM Policy Group suggests a BMI of less than 27 to be an acceptable target[13] and this might be achieved by the moderately obese diabetic, but a BMI of less than 30 may be a more realistic target for the severely obese. Once the target weight and treatment plans have been agreed by both doctor and patient they should be noted on the patient's record card and reviewed at regular intervals.

Suitable diet sheets are usually obtainable from a local hospital dietetic department and additional information may be obtained from the British Diabetic Association (BDA). *Dietary guidelines* are as follows:

1. Calorie restriction is essential but a daily intake of at least 1000 to 1200 kcal helps compliance.
2. Saturated fat intake should be reduced to less than 10% of total energy intake; mono- and polyunsaturated fatty acids may be increased so that total fat provides up to 30% of total energy.
3. Carbohydrates should be unrefined with a high fibre content and should provide 50% of total energy. This relative increase in carbohydrate is not detrimental to glycaemic control and the increase in fibre is usually beneficial.
4. Protein should generally constitute 10–15% of the daily energy intake.
5. Alcohol should be regarded as a concentrated form of calories.

Obese diabetics should therefore avoid all forms of alcohol, particularly if they also have hypertriglyceridaemia.
6. Non-caloric sweeteners such as saccharin and aspartame should be used rather than those which contain sorbitol or fructose.
7. Patients should be encouraged to divide meals evenly throughout the day and to avoid taking snacks. This prevents extremes of hunger which might lead to binge eating.
8. Selection of foods should be assisted by lists categorising them as unrestricted within reason, those which can be taken in moderation and those which should be avoided. Such lists are available from the BDA.

Group therapy for obese diabetic patients

Group sessions offer many advantages and should be seen as an important adjunct to the mini-clinic system running concurrently in the practice. Patients benefit from increased attention and from the reassurance that others share similar problems. The practice is able to structure treatment and to make effective use of staff. The increased commitment by the practice nurse is offset by a reduction in the need for individual patient follow-up in the diabetic mini-clinic.

Patients might be invited to attend group sessions on a monthly or two-monthly basis with review by the GP after six months. At the start of group treatment it is helpful for patients to keep a daily food diary. This draws attention to their own eating patterns and enables the doctor or nurse to assess approximate calorie intake. Group sessions should begin with weighing and blood glucose measurement. BMI and WHR should be calculated every six months and all results should be noted on patients' personal record cards. Teaching within the group should be carefully planned with a written syllabus to improve knowledge, compliance and control. A variety of teaching methods should be used, such as videos, role playing and demonstrations of food preparation.

Patients attending group therapy will require a structured system for longer term follow-up. Thus they might attend two revision group sessions with the nurse each year, one being combined with an appointment to see the GP in the practice diabetic clinic for an annual medical review.

Anti-obesity drugs

Many patients lose weight after their first few clinic visits but weight loss may then cease before there has been sufficient improvement in glycaemic control despite reasonable adherence to diet. Such individuals may be indentified by their carefully maintained food diaries which confirm a calorie intake of between 1000 and 1200 kcal daily. Further weight reduction may be achieved by the use of metformin, a biguanide whose anti-glycaemic action is mediated by increased insulin sensitivity and increased peripheral utilisation of glucose. The mechanism of its weight reducing action is unclear although patients often experience initial anorexia. Unfortunately, many patients also experience other effects, particularly diarrhoea, which restrict its wider use. Nevertheless, metformin remains a useful hypoglycaemic agent for the symptomatic obese diabetic particularly as the weight gain seen with the use of sulphonyureas is avoided.

For a small number of selected patients the short-term use of specific anti-obesity drugs may be helpful, provided they are used correctly as an adjunct to diet. Dexfenfluramine, which suppresses appetite by increasing central neural serotonin levels, has recently been licensed for the treatment of severe obesity. It is generally well tolerated and relatively free from side effects. In simple obesity it effectively promotes weight reduction over a one-year period[14] but as yet there are no long-term studies in obese diabetics. At the moment it is only licensed for a 12-week period of treatment. It also appears to have some intrinsic anti-diabetic activity, preliminary studies suggesting improvement in glycaemic control which is greater than might be expected from the weight loss achieved.[15] However, these findings need confirmation. Widespread use of dexfenfluramine cannot be justified but a trial might be worthwhile in a small subgroup of very obese patients who have taken part in a health promotion group for at least nine months without benefit. They should be withdrawn from the group, assessed frequently during the 12 weeks of drug treatment and then returned to the group setting for continuing follow-up.

It is possible that other anti-obesity drugs will be useful in the future. Fluoxetine, the serotonin agonist and antidepressant, reduces appetite and may have a beneficial effect on glucose tolerance. It is not yet available for the management of obesity.

Very low calorie diets.

Very low calorie diets (VLCDs) promote rapid weight loss but the long term results are disappointing. Many patients quickly regain weight immediately after stopping the diet, partly because of fluid retention, and this has a damaging effect on morale. Obese dia-

betics may be treated by VLCDs but they require specialist supervision, particularly those also taking oral hypoglycaemic drugs
where there is the risk of severe hypoglycaemia. VLCDs should not
be used in the group setting in a practice clinic.

Hyperlipidaemia

Lipoprotein abnormalities in NIDDM

Plasma lipoprotein levels in diabetic patients are affected by several
factors such as the type of diabetes, the degree of glycaemic control,
the severity and distribution of obesity, genetic influences and en-
vironmental factors such as diet, drug treatments and exercise. An
abnormality in one part of the lipoprotein system has secondary
effects elsewhere; for example a change in VLDL metabolism dis-
turbs the integrity of the VLDL-IDL-LDL cascade.

The lipoprotein profile in NIDDM is characterised by elevation
of serum VLDL triglycerides and lowering of HDL cholesterol.[16]
Hypertriglyceridaemia is frequently found in adult NIDDM
patients, the concentration of serum total and VLDL triglyceride
being 1.5 to 3 times higher than normal, depending upon glycaemic control and the degree of obesity. HDL cholesterol is
10–20% lower on average in NIDDM than controls, largely because
of a reduction in the HDL2 fraction. In contrast, the prevalence of
hypercholesterolaemia is not very different from a non-diabetic
population. Serum cholesterol commonly lies at the upper limit
of the normal range but it may be slightly elevated because tri-
glyceride-rich particles (eg VLDL) and chylomicrons also contain
significant amounts of cholesterol. The level of LDL cholesterol is
usually normal but apoprotein B is frequently elevated.

Hazards of hyperlipidaemia in diabetes

CHD is the leading cause of death in both types of diabetes and it
seems likely that the high prevalence of lipid abnormalities is contributory. In a Swedish study cholesterol was the strongest predictor
for CHD mortality in middle-aged diabetic men.[17] A positive cor-
relation has been shown between serum VLDL and vascular disease
in NIDDM and, in one study, low levels of HDL appeared to be a
marker for vascular disease but only in diabetic women.[18] The Paris
study showed plasma triglyceride, cholesterol and insulin levels
all to be risk factors for CHD mortality but the level of plasma triglyceride was the best predictor of death.[19] In the WHO multi-

national study, plasma triglyceride was also found to be a strong risk factor for CHD independent of other common risk factors.[20] Thus, in NIDDM elevated triglyceride concentrations emerge as an important independent risk factor for CHD.

Rationale for treating hyperlipidaemia in NIDDM

Treatment of moderate hyperlipidaemia in non-diabetic, normotensive subjects without overt atherogenesis reduces the incidence of cardiovascular events[21] but primary prevention trials have not shown a reduction in total mortality. Results of intervention studies have yet to be published for diabetics so the rationale for treatment is based on the results from the primary prevention studies in non-diabetics. Cardioprotection with lipid lowering agents has yet to be proven in diabetic patients but clinical judgement suggests that this group requires more active treatment than the general population. Understandably, many doctors are sceptical about the long-term benefits of relatively expensive treatments to reduce lipid concentrations. It is therefore interesting to note the parallel problem of mild hypertension. Despite the uncertain outcome from treatment of mild to moderate hypertension in non-diabetics, increasing evidence suggests that diabetics are at risk from levels of blood pressure considered normal for the non-diabetic.[22] This has led to a lower threshold for treating mild hypertension in diabetics. If this concept is also true for hyperlipidaemia it becomes important to adopt target lipid values for diabetic patients which are stricter than those for non-diabetics.

Target values for serum lipids in NIDDM

The European NIDDM policy group has agreed the target values shown in Table 1.[13] These figures represent an idealised viewpoint, justified on the basis of the high risk of CHD in diabetics. The goal

Table 1. Target values for Body Mass Index and serum lipids in diabetes as proposed by the European NIDDM Group(13).

Target	Good	Acceptable	Poor
BMI (kg/m^2)	< 25	≤ 27	> 27
Cholesterol	< 5.2	< 6.5	≥ 6.5
HDL (mmol/l)	> 1.1	≥ 0.9	< 0.9
Triglyceride (mmol/l)	< 1.7	< 2.2	≥ 2.2

for the majority of patients attending their GP clinic should be the "acceptable" target values. Although LDL cholesterol is not generally elevated in NIDDM, it has also been suggested that the target level should be substantially lower than for non-diabetics. The proposed ideal is below 2.6 mmol/l compared to 4.4 mmol/l for non-diabetics.[23] Currently, the evidence for this requirement is slender and in practice it may be very difficult to achieve.

Management of hyperlipidaemia in diabetes

Weight reduction and improved glycaemic control will correct the dyslipidaemia seen in many obese diabetics. A low fat diet and pursuit of improved glycaemic control are therefore the first steps in management. The principles of dietary strategy are essentially as described for obesity. Practices will wish to liaise with their local hosptial dietetic department to ensure that uniform advice is given across a health district. Total daily dietary fat should be reduced to 30% of the calorie intake, saturated fat being restricted to 10% of total calories and daily cholesterol to less than 300 mg. Polyunsaturates should not exceed 10% of the calories. The consequent increase in carbohydrate should be largely unrefined, ideally giving a daily fibre intake greater than 30g, but the total calorie intake must remain restricted.

NIDDM patients with poor control have the highest levels of serum triglyceride. Correction of hyperglycaemia, irrespective of method, results in a marked reduction in triglyceride and a fall in both serum and LDL cholesterol. The changes in HDL are less impressive. Strict diet may be sufficient to improve glycaemic control but in addition it may be necessary to give sulphonylureas, meformin or both. Insulin should be considered in NIDDM patients where glycaemic control fails to improve despite intensified treatment. Such a decision should be agreed with the hospital diabetologist and the patient jointly managed. Careful patient selection is essential because although insulin therapy has beneficial effects on serum lipids it may result in progressive weight gain in some cases without improvement in glycaemic control.[24]

Drug therapy of hyperlipidaemia in diabetes

Drug treatment should be considered for patients with or without good glycaemic control in whom lipid abnormalities persist despite intensive dietary efforts. Patients should recall that drug therapy is an adjunct to diet, not a substitute, and this message is easily re-

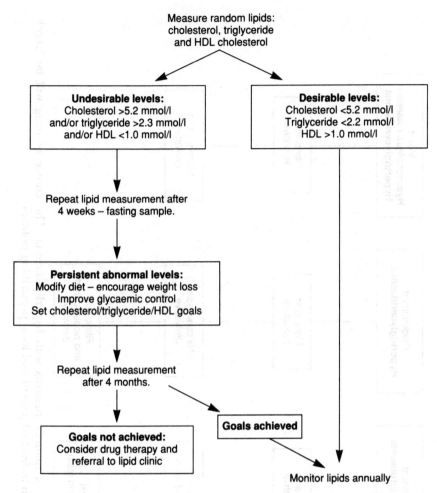

Fig. 1. Guidelines for the investigation and management of hyperlipidaemia in NIDDM patients. The proposed scheme must be adjusted to meet the individual patient's requirements.

inforced in a group setting. The decision to implement drug therapy will take account of additional risk factors such as hypertension, family history of premature vascular disease, smoking and proteinuria.

A scheme for screening and treating hyperlipidaemia in diabetic patients is illustrated in Fig. 1. Guidelines should be interpreted in the light of individual circumstances. A treatment schedule is outlined in Fig. 2. The choice of drugs will reflect local experience but fibric acid derivatives, such as bezafibrate and gemfibrozil, have proven efficacy in the treatment of dyslipidaemia associated with diabetes and are relatively free from side effects. Sustained reduc-

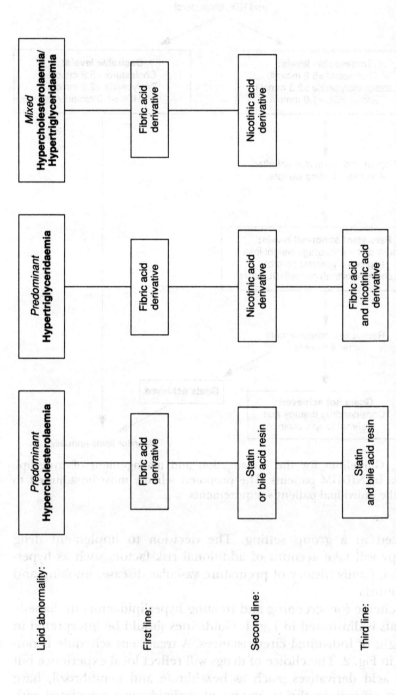

Fig. 2. Guidelines for the drug treatment of diabetic patients with hyperlipidaemia. The choice of drug will be largely dependent on the type of dyslipidaemia in an individual patient and local prescribing policies.

tions in total serum cholesterol, total triglyceride and a corresponding absolute or relative increase in HDL cholesterol may be anticipated from such agents.[25] In patients with marked hypercholesterolaemia, statin compounds (simvastatin or pravastatin) or bile acid resins (cholestyramine or colestipol) are more appropriate choices. The long term safety of the statins has yet to be confirmed and compliance may be a problem with resins which patients often find unpalatable.

Referral to hospital

The majority of patients attending their GP diabetic clinic will have moderate degrees of hyperlipidaemia which will improve with weight reduction in a group setting. Regular measurement of fasting lipids can be included in the group programme and the results discussed within the group. More severe degrees of dyslipidaemia requires additional GP involvement. A patient who fails to respond to initial measures and a first line lipid lowering drug probably requires referral to a hospital lipid or diabetic clinic.

Evaluation of care

Whatever the process adopted by the practice for managing obese hyperlipidaemic diabetic patients clinical audit will help to ensure that care is effective. Information should be collected on the number of patients attending practice nurse clinics and the number of defaulters. The percentage of patients losing a predetermined quantity of weight during a year and the number of patients attaining their target weight will be of interest. Biochemical measures might include the overall changes in glycated haemoglobin and lipid concentrations during a year and the number or percentage of patients achieving target values. Patient questionnaires will provide subjective assessment of the group strategy and enable changes to be implemented if needed. Members of the practice will need the opportunity to discuss the audit findings and contribute to proposed developments.

Summary

A scheme for the management of diabetics with obesity and hyperlipidaemia is shown in Fig. 3 and key points for successfully running a clinic system are summarised below.

1. Members of the therapeutic team will require training in counselling and communication skills.

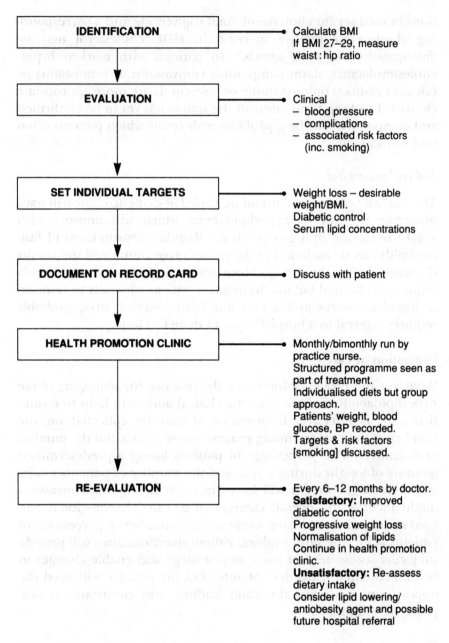

Fig. 3. A proposed scheme for the identification and management of obese, hyperlipidaemic NIDDM paients in Primary Care.

2. Diabetics should be managed in groups but dietary advice must be individualised.
3. The patient must be involved in the decision making process and agree a realistic target weight. The involvement of the family is also an advantage.
4. Regular attendance at group meetings is essential for reinforcement of diet and for exploring difficulties.
5. Continuity of care by familiar faces (practice nurse, GP and health promotion advisor) is crucial to the ultimate success of the group. The therapeutic team must meet regularly to discuss the progress of individuals within the group.
6. Short term adjuvant drug therapy may be considered in some compliant patients.
7. Group meetings should be scheduled for the most appropriate time for the members. This may require some flexibility within the practice.
8. Longer term follow-up should be planned for each patient before completion of the group programme.

Conclusion

Health promotion clinics within general practice offer an opportunity to remedy the obesity and hyperlipidaemia so common in non-insulin dependent diabetic patients. Whilst the results of intervention studies for coronary heart disease in such patients are awaited, clinical evidence argues strongly in favour of intensive treatment.

References

1. Obesity: A report of the Royal College of Physicians. *J R Coll Physicians Lond* 1983: **17**: 3–58.
2. Kissebah AH, Vydelingum N, Murray R et al. Relation of body fat distribution to metabolic complications of obesity. *J Clin Endoc Metab* 1982; **54**: 256–60.
3. WHO Measuring Obesity—classification and description of anthropometric data. 1988; WHO, Regional office for Europe, Copenhagen.
4. Rissanen A, Heliovaara M, Knekt P et al. Risk of debility and mortality due to overweight in a Finnish population. *Br Med J* 1990; **301**: 835–7.
5. Rissanen A, Heliovaara M, Knekt P *et al.* Weight and mortality in Finnish men. *J Clin Epidemiol* 1989; **42**: 781–9.
6. Manson JE, Colditz GA, Stampfer MJ et al. A prospective study of

obesity and risk of coronary heart disease in women. *N Engl J Med* 1990; **322**: 882–9.

7. Ostlund RE Jr, Staten M, Kohrt WM et al. The ratio of waist to hip circumference, plasma insulin level and glucose intolerance as independent predictors of the HDL-2 cholesterol level in older adults. *N Engl J Med* 1990; **322**: 229–34.

8. Reaven GR. Role of insulin resistance in human disease. *Diabetes* 1988; **37**: 1595–1607.

9. Joslin EP, Dublin LI, Marks HH. Studies in diabetes mellitus IV: Etiology Part II. *Am J Med Sci* 1936; **192**: 9–23.

10. UK Prospective Diabetes Study IV. Characteristics of newly presenting Type 2 diabetic patients: male preponderance and obesity at different ages. *Diabetic Med* 1988; **5**: 154–9.

11. Pearson GC, Wales JK. Dietary therapy in NIDDM. *Bailliere's Clin Endocrinol & Metab* 1988; **2**: 425–47.

12. Haddon DR, Blair ALT, Wilson EA et al. Natural History of diabetes presenting at age 40–69 years: a prospective study of the influence of intensive dietary treatment. *Quart J Med* 1986; **59**: 579–98.

13. Gries FA. Management of non-insulin dependent diabetes mellitus in Europe: a consensus statement. *Giornale Italiano di Diabetologia* 1990; **10**: 63–5.

14. Guy-Grand B, Apfelbaum M, Crepaldi G et al. International trial of long term dexfenfluramine in obesity. *Lancet* 1989; **ii**: 1142–5

15. Turtle JR, Burgess JA. Hypoglycaemic action of fenfluramine in diabetes mellitus. *Diabetes* 1973; **22**: 858–67.

16. Taskinen MR. Hyperlipidaemia in diabetes. *Bailliere's Clin Endocrinol Metab* 1990; **4**: 743–75.

17. Rosengren A, Welin L, Tsipogianni A, Wilhelmsen L. Impact of cardiovascular risk factors on coronary heart disease mortality amongst middle–aged diabetic men: a general population study. *Br Med J* 1989; **299**: 1127–31.

18. Reckless JPD, Betteridge DJ, Wu P et al. High-density and low-density lipoproteins and prevalence of vascular disease in diabetes mellitus. *Br Med J* 1978; **i**: 883–6

19. Fontbonne A, Eschwege E, Cambien F et al. Hypertriglyceridaemia as a risk factor of coronary heart disease mortality in subjects with impaired glucose tolerance or diabetes. *Diabetologia* 1989; **32**: 300–4.

20. West KM, Ahuja MMS, Bennett PH et al. The role of circulating glucose and triglyceride concentration and their interaction with other risk factors as determinants of arterial disease in nine diabetic population samples from the WHO Multinational Study. *Diabetes Care* 1983; **6**: 361–69.

21. Frick MH, Elo O, Haapa K et al. Helsinki Heart Study: primary prevention trial with gemfibrozil in middle-aged men with dyslipidaemia. *N Engl J Med* 1987; **317**: 1237–45.

22. Working Group on Hypertension in Diabetes. Statement on hypertension in diabetes. *Arch Intern Med* 1987; **147**: 830–82.

23. Garg A, Grundy SM. Management of dyslipidaemia in NIDDM. *Diabetes Care* 1990; **13**: 153–69.

24. UK Prospective Study of Therapies of Maturity-onset Diabetes.

1. Effect of diet, sulphonylurea, insulin or biguanide therapy on fasting plasma glucose and body weight over 1 year. *Diabetologia* 1983; **24**: 404–11.

25. Seviour PW, Teal TK, Richmond W, Elkeles RS. Serum lipids, lipoproteins and macrovascular disease in non-insulin dependent diabetics: a possible new approach to prevention. *Diabetic Med* 1988; **5**: 166–71.

6 | Update on long-term diabetic complications

Andrew J. M. Boulton
University of Manchester Medical School, Manchester Royal Infirmary

Complications are a function of diabetes duration and the overall level of glycaemic control.[1] Thus, it is unusual for complications to occur during the first few years of Type 1, insulin-dependent diabetes (IDDM) but the situation is entirely different for Type 2, non-insulin dependent diabetes (NIDDM) where the onset of hyperglycaemia may precede diagnosis by months or years. Long-term complications may therefore be present at the time of diagnosis of Type 2 diabetes and may even be the cause of presentation.

Early detection of complications is a fundamental part of diabetes care. Many patients will be aware of the guidelines recently published by the British Diabetic Association,[2] and will expect to be screened regularly for complications. The annual review[3] is now accepted as part of routine diabetes care in hospital and community clinics and protocols are being designed to ensure that this is done properly. Once problems have been detected they need thorough management with careful attention to detail.

Hypertension

Hypertension is not strictly a long-term complication of diabetes but it is an associated problem on a surprisingly large scale, even allowing for the effects of obesity.[4] In the United Kingdom Prospective Study of Type 2 diabetes it was found in about half of all newly diagnosed patients.[5] It should only be diagnosed if three readings on separate occasions are above 160/95–100. A large cuff should be used in obese patient with an arm circumference greater than 33 cm where the standard cuff would tend to overestimate the level of blood pressure. As with non-diabetics, the contraceptive pill, a high alcohol intake or high sodium content antacids may be contributory. Younger patients who also have complications such as retinopathy should be suspected of having diabetic nephropathy and investigated accordingly.

Weight reduction and a 'no added' salt diet may be beneficial but if blood pressure remains high, drug therapy should be considered. Although thiazide diuretics and beta-blockers remain first line anti-hypertensive drugs,[6] they should be used with caution in diabetics. Both may adversely affect serum lipids, beta-blockers may mask hypoglycaemic symptoms in insulin-treated patients and thiazides are associated with impotence and may worsen glycaemic control in Type 2 diabetics. Calcium antagonists and ACE inhibitors which do not have the metabolic disadvantages of older therapies should be considered agents of first choice in diabetic patients.[4,7] However, caution must always be exercised in the use of ACE inhibitors in older potentially arteriopathic Type 2 diabetics who might have occult renal artery stenosis.

Diabetic nephropathy

Natural history

Nephropathy occurs in both main types of diabetes, although it has been studied mostly in Type 1 diabetes. Of Type 1 diabetics, 20–40% will develop proteinuria, typically progressing to end-stage renal failure in an average of 11 years in the absence of treatment. Thus diabetic nephropathy is a major cause of renal failure in this country and accounts for a significant proportion of patients entering renal replacement programmes.

The onset of diabetic nephropathy is usually gradual and without symptoms. Incipient diabetic nephropathy is the preclinical stage in Type 1 diabetes which is predictive of later overt diabetic nephropathy. It is characterised by microalbuminuria, an increased rate of albumin excretion detectable by laboratory methods and sensitive dipsticks, but which is still below the level of detection by Albustix.

As the condition progresses to established diabetic nephropathy, proteinuria becomes intermittently positive on Albustix, but over months or years the loss of protein increases further to become continuously positive. The association with retinopathy is so strong that proteinuria in the absence of retinopathy should be investigated for other causes. Hypertension is usually present at this stage and the serum creatinine gradually rises as the glomerular filtration rate falls. If nephropathy remains undetected the first symptoms may be due to fluid retention, the nephrotic syndrome or uraemia. Renal function continues to decline at a rate fairly predictable for each individual to the point of end stage renal failure requiring dialysis or transplantation.

Screening

Routine screening for nephropathy should be carried out in all patients at least annually. This should include serum creatinine, blood pressure and urine dipstick for protein. The question of who should be screened for microalbuminuria remains controversial.[8] It should be considered in Type 1 diabetes of 5 years' duration where retinopathy and hypertension are present but where urine is albustix negative. Its detection is important as there is increasing evidence that intervention at the stage of incipient nephropathy may prevent the development of overt diabetic nephropathy. Interventions under study include ACE inhibition, strict glycaemic control, dietary protein restriction and aldose reductase inhibition.[7,9]

Management

Patients with any degree of diabetic nephropathy should be considered for early hospital referral, even if they feel well. Complex management requiring several disciplines may need to be integrated with treatments for other long-term complications. Detailed investigation including renal biopsy may be necessary to confirm the diagnosis. Excellent control of hypertension to normal or near normal levels of blood pressure and restriction of dietary protein may slow or arrest the rate of progression.[10] Patients with end-stage renal disease are best treated by renal transplantation but initially they may require chronic ambulatory peritoneal dialysis Haemodialysis is used less frequently because of problems with vascular access and because the use of heparin increases the risk of retinal haemorrhage.

Diabetic retinopathy

Screening

Although diabetes is one of the commonest causes of blindness in the working population, regular eye screening together with timely referral for treatment should prevent most cases of serious visual impairment. As in hypertension and nephropathy, symptoms do not develop until the condition is well advanced and sometimes irreversible. Risk factors for the development of retinopathy include:

- duration of diabetes;
- age at diagnosis;
- poor glycaemic control;
- presence of other long-term complications and;
- hypertension.

Diabetic retinopathy is described in detail in several excellent reviews,[3, 11-13] some of which contain colour plates.

There is continuing debate on the subject of who should screen for retinopathy. Opticians frequently examine patients' eyes and retinal cameras are used increasingly, but the diagnosis of retinopathy does rest with medical staff and screening should be performed regularly by medical staff either in practice or in hospital clinics.

All patients should have their eyes screened at diagnosis and at least annually. This should include measurement of visual acuity, with correction or pinhole if necessary, followed by assessment of lenses and fundi after pupillary dilatation with tropicamide. Exceptions to this will be patients with previous eye surgery, lens implants or narrow angle glaucoma who should not have their pupils dilated. They are likely to be under review by an ophthalmologist anyway. Those patients with no retinopathy at annual review can safely be reviewed in a year's time. Background retinopathy consisting of scattered microaneurysms and blot haemorrhages should be reviewed every 6 months.

Referral

Yellow, waxy hard exudates, readily distinguishable from drusen, are cause for concern and merit referral. This allows the ophthalmologist to assess the dynamic state of the exudates and to give timely laser treatment to the adjacent abnormally permeable vessels if necessary.

Maculopathy is characteristic of the retinopathy of Type 2 diabetes, consisting of perimacular hard exudates and macular oedema. There is the threat of rapid reduction in visual acuity which may become permanent unless treated quickly. These cases need expert assessment within a month.

Preproliferative retinopathy is characterised by cotton wool spots (soft exudates), extensive intra-retinal haemorrhages and venous tortuosity, dilatation and beading. Here again, specialist advice should be obtained within a month.

Proliferative retinopathy with new vessels on the optic disc or peripherally needs urgent referral by telephone and rubeotic glaucoma often needs immediate hospital admission.

In addition to these examples, a variety of other cases also need referral for an ophthalmological opinion. Some fundi are difficult to visualise because of severe refractive problems, keratoconus or nystagmus. There may be the possibility of glaucoma, ischaemic optic neuropathy or an incidental retinal abnormality which needs to be identified. Cataract may impair the patient's vision or pre- clude satisfactory assessment of the retina. Sudden unexplained visual loss, vascular lesions of the retina and ocular pareses always need urgent assessment. Referral to an ophthalmologist, as well as solving a clinical problem, often serves as a learning experience which increases skill and confidence.

Diabetic neuropathies

Distal sensorimotor neuropathy

The diabetic neuropathies include the relatively uncommon mononeuropathies such as carpal tunnel syndrome, foot drop and cranial nerve palsies and the much commoner polyneuropathies. Distal sensorimotor neuropathy most frequently causes clinical problems and can vary from the severely symptomatic to the completely asymptomatic insensitive foot problem. Patients with symptoms often complain of paraesthesiae, burning pains, altered temperature sensation and bedclothes hyperaesthesiae in the legs with all symptoms prone to nocturnal exacerbation. Negative symptoms include numbness and deadness and may be associated with the curious sensation of walking on air or pillows. Many people have reduced sensation to pinprick and vibration together with a degree of small muscle wasting and absent ankle reflexes. The 'painful-painless' leg is a dangerous syndrome where patients ex- perience painful symptoms but their feet are at great risk of injury because of reduced pain sensation.

Investigation and management of neuropathic disease in dia- betics has been the subject of detailed reviews.[14,15] It is certainly important to consider and exclude other possible diagnoses such as deficiency states and malignant disease. Peripheral vascular disease is the main differential diagnosis of neuropathic symptoms in the lower limb, claudication and ischaemic rest pain being associated with absent pulses, cool extremities and pallor on foot elevation.

The strategy for treating symptomatic neuropathy includes support and counselling. Glycaemic control should be improved using any method and sometimes this will mean starting Type 2 diabetics on insulin. Regular simple analgesia may give some benefit but narcotic analgesics should be avoided. A bed cradle may give nocturnal relief. If there is little improvement, imipramine 25–100 mg at night should be tried, followed by carbamazepine or phenytoin if necessary.

Proximal motor neuropathy

Proximal motor neuropathy or amyotrophy is much less common than distal sensorimotor neuropathy. The typical case is an older male Type 2 diabetic who presents with pain in the thighs, weakness and wasting which is often asymmetrical. The main differential diagnoses are carcinomatous neuropathy or spinal cord disorders. Treatment is intensive physiotherapy together with measures described for sensorimotor neuropathy.

Autonomic Neuropathy

Neuropathy may affect any area receiving autonomic innervation and although objective evidence of autonomic dysfunction is often found in diabetics, symptoms are fortunately relatively uncommon. Thus, postural hypotension, usually most marked in the morning, may only be revealed when co-existing hypertension is treated with vasodilators. Dizziness on standing tends to occur if the systolic blood pressure falls more than 30 mmHg. Gastrointestinal symptoms may need detailed investigation before a diagnosis of autonomic neuropathy is made by exclusion. Denervation of the upper gastrointestinal tract may cause anorexia, abdominal fullness, nausea and vomiting. Diabetic diarrhoea, resulting from denervation of the small bowel and sometimes aggravated by bacterial overgrowth, can be quite exhausting. There may be frequent fluid stools and faecal incontinence, typically worse at night. Disturbances of bladder function may need expert urodynamic assessment.

Impotence is another manifestation of autonomic dysfunction. Although a combination of autonomic neuropathy, vascular disease and psychological problems contribute to the aetiology in most cases, drugs such as methyl dopa, beta-blockers and thiazide diuretics may also be implicated. Iatrogenic causes should therefore be excluded before specific and sometimes invasive therapy is offered.[16]

Diabetic foot problems

Foot problems remain a major cause of morbidity and are still the commonest reason for hospital admission amongst diabetics. Early identification of those at risk of foot ulceration is one of the most important purposes of the annual review so that preventive measures can be instituted. The only equipment needed is a 128 cps tuning fork, a pin and a reflex hammer. Patients most at risk of foot problems include those with peripheral neuropathy, previous foot ulceration and co-existing foot deformities such as claw toes or hallux valgus. They are also at high risk if they have peripheral vascular disease, unilateral amputation, other diabetic complications such as blindness or nephropathy or if they are elderly, living alone and unable to care for themselves.

The neuropathic, insensitive foot may feel reassuringly warm and appear superficially healthy, but it is at great risk of ulceration. Evidence of neuropathy includes reduced sensation to any modality and absent reflexes. Patients unable to feel a vibrating tuning fork over the great toe are at risk of insensitive foot ulceration and may continue to walk despite extensive ulceration.

Effective education of these high risk patients dramatically reduces the incidence of new foot lesions.[17,18] Patients will begin to appreciate the importance of footcare if the doctor and practice nurse make a point of examining their feet and advising or demonstrating footcare at each review. A number of videos and leaflets are available to help consolidate educational messages but they are not sufficient to educate in themselves. The literature needs to be chosen carefully to avoid conflicting advice.[19] The chiropodist or local hospital clinic can give expert advice, ensuring that patients have their feet measured and that they buy broader-fitting leather shoes rather than less suitable footwear liable to cause ulceration.[20,21,22]

The patient with established foot ulceration is best referred without delay to the hospital clinic for initial diagnosis and management. This may include urgent radiology, combined antibiotic therapy, rest in hospital followed by mobilisation with pressure relieving devices and also surgery if it cannot be avoided. Once healing is well under way or complete, some or all of the subsequent care can be provided by the GP and community nurse.

Conclusion

The primary health care team has a leading role to play in the prevention, early identification and treatment of long-term diabetic complications. If prevention fails, recognition and treatment at an early stage may still avoid blindness, renal failure and amputation. According to Benjamin Franklin careful attention to detail is essential: 'A little neglect breeds mischief'.

Acknowledgements

I should like to thank Dr Lorna Young, Associate Specialist in Ophthalmology, Manchester Royal Eye Hospital, for her help with the section on retinopathy and Miss Ruth Lewis for typing the manuscript.

References

1. Godine JE. The relationship between metabolic control and vascular complications of diabetes mellitus. *Med Clin N Amer* 1988; **72**: 1271–84.
2. British Diabetic Association. What diabetic care to expect. *Diabetic Med* 1990; **7**: 554.
3. Connor H, Boulton AJM. *Diabetes in Practice.* John Wiley & Sons, Chichester, 1989.
4. Kendall MJ, Lewis H, Griffith M, Barnett AH. Drug treatment of the hypertensive diabetic. *J Hum Hypertens* 1989; **1**: 249–58.
5. Turner RC. United Kingdom prospective diabetes study III: prevalence of hypertension and hypotensive therapy in patients with newly diagnosed diabetes: a multicentre study. *Hypertension* 1985; **7 (suppl 2)**: 8–13.
6. Swales JD. First line treatment in hypertension. *Br Med J* 1990; **301**: 1172–3.
7. Boulton AJM, Gokal R. Diabetes and ACE inhibitors. *J Hum Hypertens* 1990; **4 (suppl 4)**: 63–7.
8. Rowe DJF, Dawnay A, Watts GF. Microalbuminuria in diabetes mellitus: review and recommendations for the measurement of albumin in urine. *Ann Clin Biochem* 1990; **27**: 297–312.
9. Selby JB, Fitzsimmons SC, Newman JM *et al.* The natural history and epidemiology of diabetic nephropathy. *JAMA* 1990; **263**: 1954-60.
10. Mogensen CE, Schmitz O. The diabetic kidney: from hyperfiltration and microalbuminuria to end-stage renal failure. *Med Clin N Amer* 1988; **72**: 1465–92.
11. ABC Series. The ocular examination of diabetic patients. Practical Diabetes 1985; **2(4)**: 42–3, **2(5)**: 52–4, **2(6)**: 46–8, 1986; **3**: 46–8, 102–4, 160–2, 214–6, 263, 310–2.
12. Kritzinger EE, Taylor KG. *Diabetic eye disease: an illustrated guide to diagnosis and management.* Lancaster: MTP Press Ltd, 1984.
13. Manifestations of diabetic retinopathy. In: Tasker PRW ed. *Diabetes*

(*information folder*). London: Royal College of General Practitioners, 1986.

14. Boulton AJM, Ward JD. Diabetic neuropathies and pain. *Clin Endocrinol Metab* 1986; **15**: 917–31.
15. Bays HF, Pfeifer MA. Peripheral diabetic neuropathy. *Med Clin N Amer* 1988; **72**: 1439–64
16. Gingell JC, Desai KM. Aetiology and treatment of impotence. *Practical Diabetes* 1987; **4**: 211–2, 257–63, 1988;**5**: 7–9.
17. Edmonds ME. Experience in a multidisciplinary diabetic foot clinic. In: Connor H, Boulton AJM, Ward JD eds. *The Foot in Diabetes.* Chichester: John Wiley & Sons, 1987: 121–34.
18. Boulton AJM. The diabetic foot—of neuropathic aetiology? *Diabetic Med* 1990; **7**: 852–8.
19. Day JL. Patient Education—how may recurrence be prevented? In: Connor H, Boulton AJM, Ward JD eds. *The Foot in Diabetes.* Chichester: John Wiley & Sons, 1987: 135–44.
20. Tovey FI. Care of the diabetic foot. *Practical Diabetes* 1986; **3**: 130–4.
21. Masson EA, Angle S, Roseman P et al. Foot ulcers: do patients know how to protect themselves? *Practical Diabetes* 1988; **78**:371–3.
22. Fernando DJS, Connor H, Boulton AJM. The diabetic foot 1990. *Diabetic Med* 1991; **8**: 82–5.

7 | Practical aspects of insulin therapy

A. C. Burden
Leicester General Hospital

Although insulin dependent diabetes mellitus (IDDM) has a prevalence of only 0.1%,[1] insulin-treated diabetes has a higher prevalence of up to 0.4% because of the greater number of patients with non-insulin dependent diabetes (NIDDM) who eventually come to need this form of treatment.[2,3,4] Specialist care reduces complication rates in IDDM[5,6] suggesting that such patients should remain under the supervision of diabetologists, but the position is less clear for NIDDM patients.

The first injection

IDDM is now often diagnosed at a much earlier stage than the severe weight loss, dehydration and electrolyte disturbance of typical ketoacidosis. In such cases, where the patient is ambulant and fairly fit, investigation can be restricted to a urine test and a single blood test for glucose, electrolytes and glycated haemoglobin or fructosamine. Attention can then be focused upon treatment. The patient will need to be told as sympathetically as possible that there is no alternative to insulin injections for life and that there will always be support when needed. Insulin treatment should then be started as soon as possible. Ideally the first injection should be given prior to a meal but, for training purposes, a few units could be given at any time without risk of subsequent hypoglycaemia.

With the NIDDM patient who has become poorly controlled despite maximal tablet treatment there may be lengthy discussion over weeks or months before a final decision is taken to start insulin. In these cases, insulin injections can be started at a time and place convenient to the patient. Obesity and insulin resistance may be present, causing doubt about whether insulin injections will dramatically improve either the level of glycaemic control or the long-term outcome. Such patients might be prepared to undergo a trial of insulin treatment, stopping it by agreement after a period of three months or so if there is no apparent benefit in terms of symptoms, well being or blood tests.

Other patients with badly controlled NIDDM may have evidence of marked insulin deficiency and may require insulin treatment fairly promptly. Although not strictly insulin dependent in that they may not have become ketotic, they may be extremely unwell with exhaustion, weight loss, thirst, nocturia and sometimes painful neuropathy. In some of these cases, serious consideration of insulin treatment may have been delayed unduly in the mistaken hope that it might never become necessary. Some of these patients may be frightened of 'the needle' for various reasons. They may have seen friends or family develop complications of diabetes whilst taking insulin or they may lack confidence in their ability to learn new techniques. Such patients need to start insulin as soon as possible and should be told that they will need it for life.

Patient education

Education of the diabetic starting insulin needs to be handled with great sensitivity and expertise. Ideally, any member of the diabetes care team who has a good rapport with the patient should be able to do this. Unfortunately though, many doctors and nurses are uneasy about managing this aspect of care because of lack of training.

Patients need time to familiarise themselves with the basic equipment. Simple measures like removing a new syringe from a plastic pack or opening a new insulin bottle may be awkward if one is anxious, self-conscious or inexperienced. Handling equipment will often stimulate discussion, for example about the significance of air bubbles in the syringe which do not stop the heart as many patients believe, although they do have an effect upon the amount of insulin to be injected.

Doctors and nurses advising about insulin injection, need to teach the technique as far as possible from a patient's point of view. They should be prepared to demonstrate by giving a blank injection into their own thigh, arm or anterior abdominal wall. The experienced teacher will convey the real impression that the injection is simple and easy. Reassured by this example, patients are often able to perform their own first injection using a syringe into which insulin has already been drawn up.

Injection problems

Some techniques carry the risk of intramuscular rather than subcutaneous injection of insulin, for example if the skin is stretched or if it is pinched up but allowed to drop back as the syringe needle is inserted like a dart.[7-9] In such cases, the unduly rapid absorption of insulin, particularly isophane, from the intramuscular depot may cause serious unexpected hypoglycaemia. A 45 degree approach has therefore been proposed to avoid this problem. We prefer to demonstrate how a skinfold should be pinched up and the syringe held like a pen so that the needle can be inserted perpendicular to the skin into the subcutaneous fat. Ultrasound confirms that this technique causes deposition of insulin subcutaneously rather than into muscle.

The anatomical site of insulin injection affects its rate of absorption.[10] The peak effect of any insulin occurs more rapidly after injection into the anterior abdominal wall or arm compared to the leg. These differences can be exploited to advantage in different situations. For example, injection of a quick acting insulin into the abdomen is highly convenient in a restaurant just prior to a meal. However, as most people rely upon consistency and predictability of absorption we recommend the use of one anatomical site, the leg, most of the time.

Good glycaemic control is dependent upon good injection technique. The common problem of lipohypertrophy needs to be avoided as repeated insulin injection into a small subcutaneous area has an adverse effect upon the consistency of insulin absorption. Injection into a lipohypertrophied area delays absorption[12] and chance injection into the zone of increased vascularity surrounding the abnormal area might enhance absorption. We therefore suggest that patients inject over a wide area of each thigh using an imaginary square grid system, from a hand's width above the knee to half a hand's width below the groin creaseline. The medial limit of the injection sites should be the trouser creaseline and the lateral limit the furthermost point which can be conveniently seen and pinched up. Patients should begin with one leg, inject into the lower thigh, work upwards with each consecutive injection and on reaching the upper limit restart at the bottom more medially or laterally. The process should be repeated until all of the imaginary grid squares have been used once. The process is then repeated on the other leg before alternating back again.[11]

Conclusion

Most patients soon realise that injecting insulin is fairly straightforward compared to the real challenge of managing their own diabetes in the long term. Despite their willingness to learn, they can only assimilate a limited amount of information at any given time. Education should therefore be restricted initially to simple rules of safety. Subsequently, they can be taught about the effects of mood, stress, food, temperature and exercise on control and the impact of control itself on diabetes. Algorithms abound for the adjustment of insulin, but these should be individualised according to circumstances.

References

1. Samanta A, Burden AC, Jones GR, et al. Prevalence of insulin dependent diabetes mellitus in Asian children. *Diabetic Med* 1987; **4**: 65–7.
2. Gatling W, Houston AC, Hill RD. The prevalence of diabetes mellitus in a typical English community. *J R Coll Physicians Lond* 1985; **19**: 248–50.
3. Mather HM, Keen H. The Southall Diabetes Survey: prevalence of known diabetes in Asians and Europeans. *Br Med J* 1985; **291**: 1081–4.
4. Waugh NR, Jung RT, Newton RW. The Dundee prevalence study of insulin-treated diabetes: intervals between diagnosis and start of insulin therapy. *Diabetic Med* 1989; **6**: 346–50.
5. McNally PG, Burden AC, Swift PGF, Walls J, Hearnshaw JR. The prevalence and risk factors associated with the onset of diabetic neuropathy in juvenile onset (insulin-dependent) diabetes diagnosed under the age of 17 years in Leicestershire 1930–1985. *Quart J Med* 1990; **76**: 831–44.
6. Hearnshaw JR, McNally PG, Swift PGF, Burden AC. Factors associated with the development of diabetic retinopathy in juvenile onset (under 16 years) insulin-dependent diabetes. *Diabetes Res Clin Pract* 1988; **5 (suppl)**: S298.
7. Spraul M, Chauteleau E, Koumoulidou J, Berger M. Subcutaneous or non-subcutaneous injection of insulin. *Diabetes Care* 1988; **11**: 733–6.
8. Frid A, Linden B. Where do lean diabetics inject their insulin? A study using computed tomography. *Br Med J* 1986; **292**: 1638.
9. Frid A, Gunnarson R, Gunter P, Linden B. Effects of accidental intramuscular injection on insulin absorption in IDDM. *Diabetes Care* 1988; **11**: 41–5.
10. Houtzagers CMGJ. Subcutaneous insulin delivery: present status. *Diabetic Med* 1989; **6**: 754–61.
11. Burden AC, Jones GR, Blandford RL. Insulin injection technique and diabetic control. *Pract Diabetes* 1984; **1**: 10–13.
12. Thow JC, Johnson AB, Marsden S, Taylor R, Home PD. Morphology of palpably abnormal injection sites and effects on absorption of isophane (NPH) insulin. *Diabetic Med* 1990; **7**: 795–9.

8 | Starting insulin at home

Diana Piper
North Devon District Hospital, Barnstaple, Devon

Domiciliary care of diabetic patients was under way many years ago.[1] More recently, with stronger emphasis on integrated teamwork and with the availability of diabetes specialist nurses there has been a greater readiness to start insulin in the home.[2,3]

Patient profiles

If we look at the diabetic population we can get a general idea of which patients are likely to start insulin at home. Between a fifth and a quarter of all diabetics are insulin dependent (IDDM). Increased awareness and prompt investigation means that many of these young people are diagnosed well before the stage of severe metabolic decompensation. They are therefore relatively fit, although symptomatic, and do not need hospital admission as long as their serum electrolytes are satisfactory and provided insulin can be started immediately at home.

Nearly a third of IDDM patients are diagnosed above the age of 30, sometimes in late life, and although presentation may be as dramatic as in the young, progression to insulin dependence is often gradual.[4] These late presenting IDDM patients are sometimes initially mistaken as being non-insulin dependent diabetics (NIDDM).[5] They are usually unwell with hyperglycaemic symptoms, weight loss and ketonuria, indicating marked insulin deficiency. They may have a first degree family history of IDDM.[6] They are only too ready to start insulin as soon as it can be organised and any misgivings about this form of treatment resolve as they regain their lost energy.

It is quite safe to start selected children on insulin at home but most centres in the UK are unwilling to do this, partly because the tempo of disease is often much faster than in adults and very close supervision may suddenly become necessary. With these cases, a short admission to hospital may give parents a brief respite to attune themselves to the idea that their child now has a lifelong condition needing careful home management. Even so, an effective domiciliary service allows such children to be discharged soon, perhaps the day after starting insulin, so that their main educational programme can still take place at home.

The choice between insulin and tablets for NIDDM patients is often difficult[7] but in practice about a quarter of patients will become insulin-treated.[8,9] Statistically then, a person starting insulin at home is just as likely to be an elderly NIDDM patient as a much younger person prone to ketosis. In the UK, it is unusual for insulin to be used in primary diet failure as a direct alternative to drug therapy. It is more likely to be considered in patients whose diabetes remains poorly controlled despite maximum doses of tablets. The exact criteria remain flexible, but if one were aiming for normoglycaemia 90% of NIDDM patients would need a trial of insulin after 5 years' tablet treatment. The UK Prospective Diabetes Study may clarify these points by showing whether it is better to lower blood glucose using insulin or tablets.

Obese NIDDM patients present a particular dilemma which can only be resolved on an individual basis. One view is that insulin treatment should be avoided because insulin resistance results in large insulin requirements and further weight gain without necessarily improving glycaemic control.[10] The contrary view is that one should simply use whatever doses of insulin are necessary.[11] Insulin has an important place in the temporary treatment of NIDDM patients during episodes of poor control precipitated by intercurrent illness. It may also help in the treatment of certain diabetic complications such as amyotrophy or acute painful neuropathy.

Insulin is sometimes needed for a while in diabetes induced by steroid treatment for conditions like vasculitis or severe asthma. Occasionally it may improve the quality of remaining life in terminal neoplastic disease such as carcinoma of the pancreas. Patients are often grateful when they can be treated in their home environment with continuing support from relatives and hospice nurses. Of gestational diabetics, 10–15% are likely to need insulin[12] and if this is started at home there is minimal disruption to the rest of the family.

Setting up

Starting insulin treatment at home can only be successful if the professional environment is favourable. This requires a clear definition of roles, an accepted chain of responsibility and excellent lines of communication. Our own policy is for every patient to be assessed by a consultant, on the day of referral if necessary. The diabetes specialist nurse attends that consultation, either to meet the patient for the first time or to continue a relationship which may have started some time before in the patient's home at the request of the GP. Objectives of treatment are defined, the types, timing and initial doses of insulin are prescribed and a home monitoring policy is agreed. The telephone network is noted so that patients can be contacted or make contact at any time. This information is then communicated by telephone to the GP and practice nurse and confirmation is sent by letter. The diabetes specialist nurse then arranges when she will visit the patient's home to start the treatment.

Some NIDDM patients will be well prepared for insulin treatment because of previous discussions. They will already have an extensive background knowledge of diabetes provided by their diabetes specialist nurse and practice nurse. In addition, at first mention of the possibility of insulin treatment, perhaps weeks or months before, they will have given themselves a trial injection.[13]

The situation is more demanding with the newly diagnosed insulin dependent diabetic. Patient and family may be emotionally confused and respond more to the warmth and support of non-verbal signals than to any information given at an intellectual level. Although they should take a major part in policy making, patients often acquiesce to initial decisions made on their behalf by the professional staff, preferring to delay more active involvement until they can think clearly. In such cases, they are started on insulin the same day, with the involvement of any family member who can help, either in the clinic or at home. In addition to the basic injection technique, they are also taught about the recognition and treatment of hypoglycaemia. The rest of the educational and counselling programme proceeds over the next few weeks at a rate suited to their learning capacity.

Insulin strategies

Initial emphasis is upon safety and simplicity then, over a period of time, the insulin strategy is individualised for each person. As a general rule our patients are first taught to use plastic disposable syringes and insulin bottles rather than pen injectors so that they always have this standard method to fall back on. The first few injections are supervised at home until the method is accurate. Some weeks later, when basic technique is sound, the available pen injectors are demonstrated so that they can be tried. Sometimes the most preferred pen may not be compatible with the most preferred insulin cartridges but hopefully this problem will be overcome in the future by a more patient-orientated industry. Patients are reminded that although pen injectors may increase convenience, they do not necessarily improve glycaemic control.[14]

Most of our IDDM patients are started on a twice daily premixed insulin containing 30% soluble and 70% isophane. This is quickly understood by most patients, mixing errors are eliminated and dose adjustments do not need too much thought. Glycaemic control is usually as good as if the two separate insulins are drawn up to an individual formula. Over the next few weeks the limitations of this treatment are explored so that it can be adapted to life style. In some cases the twice daily pattern of injections is continued but the ratio of insulins in the mixture is changed. For example, troublesome hypoglycaemia mid morning might resolve and blood glucose before the evening meal might still remain satisfactory with a change in the formulation of the morning insulin to 20% soluble and 80% isophane. In other cases there is a need for the flexibility of an intensified insulin regimen: soluble insulin three times daily before meals with an isophane insulin before bed. Again, patients need to realise that the multiple injection regimen is not primarily a way of improving glycaemic control.

Policies for treating NIDDM with insulin tend to vary, from relief of hyperglycaemic symptoms in some cases to achievement of near normoglycaemia in others. It has been suggested that overnight insulin is a physiological treatment for NIDDM, a long-acting insulin before bed suppressing the abnormally high basal rate of hepatic glucose production.[15] Like others,[6] we find that a single injection of a long acting insulin before bed is not usually sufficient to prevent daytime hyperglycaemia in NIDDM patients who have become badly controlled on tablets. A morning injection is often required as well, but elderly people may become confused if it is a different type of insulin from the evening injection. In consequence, many of our NIDDM patients eventually become happily stabilised on twice daily premixed insulins.

Insulin dosage

There is less mystique to insulin doses than many people believe, but during the period of rapid adjustment maximum safety is achieved if the patient, the specialist nurse and the consultant or GP maintain daily contact. To the wasted insulin dependent diabetic any injected insulin is better than none. We often start with as little as four units twice daily and then quickly increase the doses each day. At the end of the first week such a patient might be on perhaps 20 to 36 units of a 30/70 insulin mixture in the morning and 10 to 18 units in the evening. Thereafter, doses might gradually change according to compensatory overeating, the effect of the 'honeymoon period' and other factors, but adjustment would be dominated by results of blood glucose tests. The NIDDM patient with insulin resistance might need much more insulin but doses would also be very dependent upon the ability to adhere to a diet.[16]

The 'rule of thirds' has sometimes been recommended as a way of sighting up on doses in a twice daily insulin regimen. This suggests that in any day two thirds of the total dose should be given as an isophane and one third as a soluble insulin. Because of the endogenous diurnal variation in insulin sensitivity, two thirds of the total insulin dose should be given in the morning and one third in the evening. In practice, premixed insulins containing 30% soluble and 70% isophane can simply be used at twice the dose in the morning compared to the evening. There may be problems with this simple formula but it is a useful starting point. Thus, in a patient starting insulin at home, after the initial injections which will tend to be low dose and roughly equal in the morning and evening, the morning dose should be increased at a faster rate than the evening dose. An exception to this is the elderly patient who might become confused and get the doses the wrong way round. In such cases it is safer if the morning and evening doses are identical and also low enough to eliminate any possibility of hypoglycaemia.

Various formulae also exist for converting from a twice to a four times daily insulin regimen. It is prudent to reduce the total dose at times of change, accepting a few days of slightly worse control rather than risking severe hypoglycaemia. In practice it should be possible to give 40–60% of the total daily insulin dose as the evening isophane, the rest being divided into thirds for injection as the soluble before each meal. The dose of evening insulin is adjusted to give the best blood glucose on waking whilst avoiding nocturnal hypoglycaemia and attention is then focused on individualising preprandial doses.

Monitoring

Strategies for self monitoring have to be realistic so that patients can comply and also respond appropriately to the messages conveyed by their tests. Initial testing needs to be intensive. If possible, capillary blood glucose measurements should be performed several times daily for the first few weeks. Some patients cannot cope with this, but they are prepared to do frequent urine tests for the first week or so, after which they are able to convert to blood glucose testing.

As glycaemic control settles down a preferred testing strategy should emerge which should then be formalised so that patients feel at ease with it and not guilty. Young patients might do blood glucose testing twice daily at different times on two or three days a week with additional tests for special circumstances such as sport, driving or exams. In practice, the outcome from different testing routines is very similar.[17] We are always prepared to demonstrate a range of meters which patients can borrow for a trial period before making a final decision to buy one. However, paired testing in which capillary blood glucose measurements are validated by the laboratory[18] shows that patients are often sufficiently accurate to read test strips visually without the need for a meter. The weak point in their strategy is often the failure to adjust insulin once their blood glucose is known.

Although blood glucose testing is extremely important in maintaining good glycaemic control some patients express a strong preference for urine testing, especially farmers, mechanics and other workers whose fingers are at greater than average risk of infection. These people may wish to do regular urine tests and use blood tests as a way of solving specific problems. Some patients simply refuse to do blood tests but may be prepared to do urine tests several times daily and before bed. They can achieve excellent glycaemic control by aiming to be completely free from glycosuria throughout the day whilst at the same time reducing their insulin slightly if they get hypoglycaemic symptoms. For older patients, twice weekly urine tests, before breakfast and before bed, may be the most convenient. Occasional blood tests can also be performed to clarify the position at certain times of the day, for example if a headache following afternoon somnolence suggests the possibility of hypoglycaemia.

Merits of home stabilisation

Diabetes care is most successful if it is adapted to patients' life styles, fitting in with habitual eating, exercise and work patterns. Within the familiar home environment patients are able to look upon their diabetes as a way of life rather than a hospital or general practice based disease process. They are often able to relax and absorb educational messages to which they would be impervious in the unfamiliar atmosphere of a clinic or diabetes centre. Avoiding hospital admission, as well as saving money[3] allows patients to continue at work, to look after their children and to enjoy their hobbies. The elderly are less likely to become confused. Family members can also learn about diabetes and can express their involvement in constructive ways. There is also greater depth to the quality of the therapeutic relationship with the visiting nurse who is perceived as a friend and a guest. If needed, the specialist nurse can continue to act as a key worker, involving and liaising with other carers such as the community nursing sister, practice nurse, GP, health visitor and social worker. There is opportunity for direct liaison between the hospital and the primary care team if the specialist nurse and the GP visit by arrangement at the same time. GPs are sometimes uncertain about adjusting insulin[19] so seeing the process in action in their own patients can increase confidence.

Elderly patients are often grateful for detailed advice on subjects which are important to them but which would seem trivial in a clinic, such as whether insulin should be kept downstairs in the refrigerator or upstairs in the bathroom. Functional assessment of tremulous or partially sighted patients may lead to effective solutions such as the provision of alignment jigs for drawing up insulin, low vision aids, better lighting conditions and help from relatives or neighbours. With careful environment management it should be possible for the great majority of elderly insulin-treated diabetics to manage without regular visits from district nurses.

Next steps

Once patients are satisfied with their progress and have learnt how to look after their diabetes, they can be given the opportunity to become increasingly self-sufficient. This is important for morale and makes them feel that they are not over-dependent upon health care. Even so, further provision is made in various ways. Links are strengthened between the patient and the primary health care team and an appointment is also made for the hospital diabetic clinic, usually three months after starting insulin but sometimes earlier if there are problems such as insulin oedema or worsening retino-pathy. Those who wish it are put in touch with local self-help groups. Diabetes specialist nurses maintain regular telephone contact to offer counselling and support and also visit on request.

References

1. Walker JB. Fieldwork of a diabetic clinic. *Lancet* 1953; **ii**: 445–7.
2. Wilson RM, Clarke P, Barkes H, Heller SR, Tattersall RB. Starting insulin treatment as an outpatient: report of 100 consecutive patients followed for a year. *JAMA* 1986; **256**: 877–80.
3. Tomlinson S. The aims of diabetes care. *This volume.*
4. Kilvert A, Fitzgerald MG, Wright AD, Nattrass M. Clinical characteristics and aetiological classification of insulin-dependent diabetes in the elderly. *Quart J Med* 1986; **60**: 865–72.
5. Wilson RM, Van der Minne P, Deverill I et al. Insulin dependence: problems with the classification of 100 consecutive patients. *Diabetic Med* 1985; **2**: 167–72.
6. Tattersall RB, Scott AR. When to use insulin in the maturity onset diabetic. *Postgrad Med J* 1987; **63**: 859–64.
7. Martin DB. Type 2 diabetes: insulin versus oral agents. *N Engl J Med* 1986; **314**: 1314–5.
8. Nabarro JDNN. Diabetes in the United Kingdom: a personal series. *Diabetic Med* 1991; **8**: 59–68.
9. Gatling W, Houston AC, Hill RD. The prevalence of diabetes mellitus in a typical English community. *J R Coll Physicians Lond* 1985; **19**: 248–50.
10. Boden G. Treatment strategies for patients with non-insulin-dependent diabetes mellitus. *Am J Med* 1985; **979 (Suppl 2B)**: 23–6.
11. Lardinois CK, Liu GC, Reaven GM. Glyburide in non-insulin-dependent diabetes: its therapeutic effect in patients with disease poorly controlled by insulin alone. *Arch Int Med* 1985; **145**: 1028–32.
12. Barss VA. Diabetes in pregnancy. *Med Clins N Amer* 1989; **73**: 685–700.
13. Burden AC. Practical aspects of insulin therapy. *This volume.*
14. Houtzagers CMGJ, Visser AP, Berntzen PA et al. Multiple daily insulin injections improve self-confidence. *Diabetic Med* 1989; **6**: 512–9.
15. Turner RC, Phillips MA, Ward EA. Ultralente basal insulin regimens—clinical applications, advantages and disadvantages. *Acta Med Scand* 1983; **671**: 75–86.
16. Reaven GM. Beneficial effect of moderate weight loss in older patients with NIDDM poorly controlled with insulin. *J Am Geriatric Soc* 1985; **33**: 93–5.
17. Gordon D, Semple CG, Paterson KR. Do different frequencies of self-monitoring of blood glucose influence control in Type 1 diabetic patients? *Diabetic Med* 1991; **8**: 679–82.
18. Paisey RB, Bradshaw P, Hartog M, West P. Home monitoring of blood glucose using filter paper strips. *Br Med J* 1979; **ii**: 1509.
19. Marsden P, Grant J. The learning needs in diabetes of general practitioners. *Diabetic Med* 1989; **7**: 69–73.

9 | Good control or a happy life?

K. G. M. M. Alberti

Department of Medicine, University of Newcastle upon Tyne

Ideally the treatment for any chronic condition should be designed to maintain as near normal a quality of life as possible. With this in mind, we need to look at the advantages and disadvantages of good control of blood glucose, to see whether attainment of good control need necessarily have a negative impact on the daily life of diabetic patients.

Aims of treatment

There are two main aims of treatment for diabetes. The first is to allow as normal a daily life as possible without symptoms whilst at the same time avoiding acute complications such as ketoacidosis, hypoglycaemia and infection. The second is to prevent or delay the long-term specific complications of diabetes including micro-angiopathy (retinopathy, nephropathy), cataract and neuropathy and to decrease the excess morbidity and mortality from macro-vascular disease.

Initially, in 1921, it was felt that replacement of insulin alone would achieve these goals, but by the 1930s it was clear that neither of these aims was being met. In the ensuing three decades the first goal was more nearly achieved, but again complications were rampant. In the 1970s and 1980s a growing belief developed that it would be necessary to achieve sustained normoglycaemia to avoid the long-term problems of diabetes. This was built on the classic reports of Pirart[1] and Job *et al*[2] although there were many defects in their studies. However, the development of continuous sub-cutaneous insulin infusion by Pickup *et al*[3] allowed the attainment of near-normoglycaemia. This technique was employed by several groups to show that good glycaemic control over a 2 to 5 year period could arrest the progression of early retinopathy and nephro-pathy.[4-6] We have therefore now reached a situation where it is assumed that normoglycaemia is the primary goal of treatment for both insulin dependent (IDDM) and non-insulin dependent diabetes mellitus (NIDDM).

Balancing advantages and disadvantages

The putative advantages of good glycaemic control include symptom relief, a feeling of well-being and avoidance of acute complications. For this set of goals the acceptable limits of glycaemia are relatively broad, perhaps 3 to 11, or 12 mmol/l. By contrast, the 'normoglycaemia' necessary to prevent long-term complications assumes blood glucose levels of 3 to 7 or 8 mmol/l, although we still do not know for sure what the upper level of glycaemia should be to avoid chronic complications.

Personal freedom

There would be no objection to striving for normoglycaemia if there were no disadvantages in so doing. Yet this quest requires many compromises which encroach upon personal freedom to the point where many people with IDDM find life very restricted. A fixed amount of insulin is injected, usually twice daily, which then requires careful balancing against food and exercise. A major problem arises because of the absorption pharmacokinetics of subcutaneous insulin.[7] Absorption is slow even for rapid acting insulins and necessitates the taking of snacks two to three hours after main meals. Even with a rigid regimen, glycaemic control is imperfect because of the large day-to-day variation in the rate of insulin absorption. In addition, no insulin preparation gives the smooth constant delivery of insulin throughout the night which occurs with physiological insulin secretion.

Some of this rigidity of lifestyle can be avoided by the use of multiple injections of short acting insulin with an intermediate acting insulin at bedtime. If patients monitor blood glucose on a regular basis the doses of insulin can be modified according to current glucose levels and intended food intake. Timing of meals and insulin injections are less critical, so much greater flexibility of life style becomes possible. Injection pens have greatly facilitated these multiple injection regimens. Even so, because frequent blood glucose self monitoring is necessary the IDDM person cannot forget about diabetes.

Hypoglycaemia

The other great concern of the IDDM patient is hypoglycaemia. The incidence has increased with the greater emphasis on attaining normoglycaemia so that at least 10% of patients will have one severe episode of hypoglycaemia per year.[8] This is partly due to the erratic pharmacokinetics of injected insulin, with nocturnal hypoglycaemia posing a particular problem. Lessened warning of impending hypoglycaemia also appears more prevalent, partly due to prolonged spells of normoglycaemia or near hypoglycaemia.[9] Hypoglycaemia is also a probable component of the recently popularised 'death in bed' syndrome,[10] which although rare is nonetheless a frightening prospect, particularly for those living alone.

Similar, although less severe, problems arise in NIDDM patients. Hypoglycaemia occurs in many subjects taking sulphonylureas, notably the longer acting preparations, chlorpropamide and glibenclamide. This is a particular problem in the elderly causing many hospital admissions, and indeed deaths.[11] One suspects that mild hypoglycaemia is also common in the elderly where symptoms may be attributed to the confusion that can occur with ageing.

Monitoring

Intensive monitoring is also a negative aspect of striving for good control. This is especially true for young IDDM subjects, who may make up many of their results to please the doctor but cannot face repeated finger-pricking in practice.[12] Urine testing is also found to be unpleasant by many elderly patients.

Diet

Dietary restrictions or dietary changes are also a potential problem. They can lead to great frustration and a sense of guilt, although current education should prevent this because of greater flexibility.

Hyperinsulinaemia

Finally, it has been suggested that hyperinsulinaemia may be a cause of atheroma.[13] In order to achieve good glycaemic control with peripheral subcutaneous insulin therapy in IDDM, it is inevitable that peripheral hyperinsulinaemia should occur.[14] In NIDDM where insulin resistance is a dominant component of the disorder, hyperinsulinaemia is also common and may be worsened by treatment.

Nonetheless the risk of hyperinsulinaemia causing damage is still unproven.

Conclusion

The advantages of striving for good glycaemic control must be weighed against the disadvantages. Definitive proof of the benefits of good control must await the outcome of the American Diabetes Control and Complications Trial and the UK Prospective Diabetes Study. In the interim, however, the benefits appear large. Intensive patient education will undoubtedly help to avoid many of the disadvantages. One must titrate measures to achieve good control to such a point for each individual where the putative advantages still clearly outweigh the problems. Pushing for tight control at all cost is as unwarranted as a nihilistic approach to any form of good control. In elderly subjects the targets will be less stringent but, again, each case must be considered individually.

It is indeed possible for an individual to have both good control *and* a happy life, but this is not universal and requires considerable effort on the part of both the health care team and the patient.

References

1. Pirart J. Diabetes mellitus and its degenerative complications: a prospective study of 4400 patients observed between 1947 and 1973. *Diabete Metab* 1977; **3**: 97–107, 173–82, 245–56.
2. Job D, Eschwege E, Guyot-Argenton C, Aubry JP, Tchobroutsky G. Effect of multiple daily insulin injections on the course of diabetic retinopathy. *Diabetes* 1976; **25**: 463–9.
3. Pickup JC, Keen H, Parsons JA, Alberti KGMM. Continuous subcutaneous insulin infusion: good blood glucose control for up to four days. *Diabetologia* 1979; **16**: 385–9.
4. Lauritzen T, Frost-Larsen K, Larsen HW, Deckert T, The Steno Study Group. Two years' experience with continuous subcutaneous insulin infusion in relation to retinopathy and neuropathy. *Diabetes* 1985; **34 (Suppl 3)**: 74–9.
5. Kroc Collaborative Study Group. Diabetic retinopathy after two years of intensified insulin treatment. Follow-up of the Kroc collaborative study. *JAMA* 1988; **260**: 37–41.
6. Dahl-Jorgensen K. Near-normoglycaemia and late diabetic complications. The Oslo Study. *Acta Endocrinologica* 1987; **115 suppl 284**: 1–36.
7. Home PD, Thow JC. Insulin injection therapy. In: Alberti KGMM, Krall LP, eds. *Diabetes Annual* 5. Amsterdam: Elsevier, 1990: 152–65.
8. Cryer PE, Binder C, Bolli GB, et al. Hypoglycaemia in IDDM. *Diabetes* 1989; **38**: 1193-9.
9. Amiel SA, Tamborlane SV, Simonson DC, Sherwin RS. Defective

glucose counterregulation after strict glycaemic control of insulin-dependent diabetes mellitus. *N Engl J Med* 1987; **316**: 1376–83.

10. Campbell IW. Dead in bed syndrome: a new manifestation of nocturnal hypoglycaemia. *Diabetic Med* 1991; **8**: 3–4.
11. Ferner RE, Neil HAW. Sulphonylureas and hypoglycaemia. *Br Med J* 1988; **296**: 949–50.
12. Petranyi G, Burrin JM, Alberti KGMM. What is wrong with home blood glucose monitoring? Use of memory meters in problem patients in a diabetes outpatient clinic. *Diab Nutr Metab* 1988; **1**: 119–23.
13. Robertson DA, Hale PJ, Nattrass M. Macrovascular disease and hyperinsulinaemia. *Bailliere's Clin Endocrinol Metab* 1988; **2**: 407–24.
14. Alberti KGMM. Insulin treatment and diabetes: half a century of therapeutic misadventure. In: Tunbridge WMG ed. *Advanced Medicine.* London: Pitman Medical 1981: 1–13.